"Stories are how we make sense of the world. Stories are how we find meaning in the face of life's travails. In this collection, hospice nurse Sharon White shares stories born of the wisdom of her many years spent in the homes and at the bedside of persons nearing the end of life. Readers, be they patients, family members or health care professionals, will find that the stories ring true and will provide them with guidance when they too encounter the challenges that arise near the end of life."

Paul Bascom, MD FACP, OHSU, Palliative Medicine and Comfort Care Team

———

"Do you find yourself wondering about your own or your loved ones' end of life care? This book explores the journey of a compassionate hospice nurse as she grapples with many of the questions we all face. You will both laugh and cry as you enter the world of the author. The book is creatively sprinkled with thoughtful poetry for reflection. I recommend this book to anyone in search of the truth about dying and about hospice."

Eddy Marie Crouch, Licensed Clinical Social Worker

———

"Sharon has a beautiful way of getting to the truth of life. She weaves the many interesting and "very real" stories of her patients' lives in an example of what it truly means to be present with the dying. Her stories explain how to support all those connected with the dying, how to be with a less than ideal situation, how to be open and raw, how to be filled with gratitude and how to be present in the world of the dying. These stories are authentic. Sharon acts and speaks bravely from her heart. Your perception of death will change after reading this book."

Teresa Looper, R.N., B.S.N., C.P.H.N., co-worker and supervisor of Portland Providence Hospice

"As a former Hospice Administrator and nurse it was my privilege to be asked to read Whose Death Is It, Anyway?. I was fortunate enough to have been Sharon's supervisor and have the opportunity to hear her patient summaries in our Monday morning rituals. I was always deeply touched by her communication skills. This book is one that really touches the "Heart of Hospice."

"I am delighted that Sharon is using these stories to reach out to patients facing death, to families and to all health care providers. This book can be a very useful tool for education for all interested in the dying process."

Barbara McEachern R.N. Former Administrator, Director of Nurses, Willamette Falls Hospice

Whose Death Is It, Anyway?
A Hospice Nurse Remembers

By Sharon White, R.N., B.S.N

Publisher's Information

EBookBakery Books
www.ebookbakery.com

Cover design: Karl Gillespie
www.diversitydesign.com

Author contact: sharinjoy2003@hotmail.com

ISBN 978-1-938517-31-0

To ensure confidentiality of those I served, names have been changed.
I took the opportunity to inform and gain permission, when possible,
to include their story from most persons. Composite stories have been
included in an attempt to avoid major repetition.

How does love greet Death?

With a hug
a kiss
and
a tear.

Sharon White

ACKNOWLEDGMENTS

I wish to thank members of my Chrysalis writing group for giving encouragement when needed and critique with each reading. I appreciated each comment and especially the reading of the manuscript by Linda Appel, Alice Lynn and Pat Lichen. I am eternally grateful to my professional peers who encouraged me when I was working with them, volunteered to read the stories and made suggestions regarding content of the stories. I'd like to mention a few of these wonderful hospice workers: Anne LaBorde L.C.S.W., Teresa Looper, **R.N., B.S.N., C.P.H.N.**

Dedication

I wish to dedicate this book to Paula Gillespie who with her family, daughter and two sons fought ovarian cancer bravely. During this process she insisted on reading and commenting on my entire manuscript. Her story appears in the book in the chapter—Goodbye to a Friend.

I would be remiss if I didn't acknowledge all the families I refer to in this book. It is indeed a brave family who travels the journey with their loved one. I thank you for the gifts you have given me. I certainly gained much more than I gave.

TABLE OF CONTENTS

FOREWORD

Responses to dying and the death of a loved one are as different as our individual personalities. Though the goal is acceptance and to help the patient let go, the journey to that end is varied and often filled with obstacles. When medical resources for curing have been exhausted; when a doctor has used the words: "I'm sorry but here is nothing more we can do. I'm referring hospice in to help," that's when patients and families turn to hospice supports.

At this point, hospice becomes a copilot, but the patient, when able, remains the driver. It's the disease itself that has the foot on the pedal. The hospice team will direct the patient's care, but in doing so, they will remain sensitive to the needs, expectations and physical symptoms of the dying and be attentive to the concerns of his or her support system. It is a time of many themes: acceptance, forgiveness, gratitude and surrender. It is also a time of challenges including the need to balance the patient's decline with the medications used for pain control.

Whose death is it, anyway?

Ultimately the patient's death echoes thoughts of our own mortality. We all know that it is not a question of IF death will happen to us. It is a question of when, where, how and of who will be present when our time comes. Try as we might, no one gets out of life alive and no doctor can make a patient immortal. The question becomes, what will our challenges be when our time comes?

The stories in Whose Death Is It, Anyway? are tributes to the brave: the patients, their families and the team of professionals who continue to be present for the final journey. As you read them, I'm sure you will find reason to laugh, cry and even identify with my patients and with the families who love and support them. I acknowledge and am grateful for the patient, the family and my coworkers. I have gained much insight from all of them.

Sharon White, R.N., B.S.N, 2014

PART ONE

Denial

DEATH ON ADMISSION

"I just got a call from a physician," my supervisor says interrupting my paperwork. "He said Stella's family wants hospice immediately. They think she's dying right now. He's signed the orders. Since she lives in your area, could you do the admission visit?"

After two deaths in two work days, I think I need a rest. But in the interest of the family, doctor and most of all the patient, I nod. "What's her diagnosis?" I ask, knowing that, regardless of the diagnosis, end stage requires packing the equivalent of five visits into one. This type of admission, if indeed she is close to death, is labor-intensive and could take as long as three or four hours. The process is always ladened with heavy emotions: denial, guilt, resentment and a host of other feelings. I know I'm wrung out when I finish one of these challenges.

"End-Stage Lung Cancer—with maximum chemo and radiation therapy. This family sounds nice, but scared. Her son says his mom has fought very hard but now she wants to be allowed to die." My supervisor tries to smile. "I know it's been a hard week for you. You can pick up the necessary medications in about fifteen minutes. I'll call the family and tell them you're on your way. Is that okay?"

I signal my assent and take a deep breath—no time to give in to fatigue.   Once on the road, I review my mental checklist, preparing for what might be ahead of me. I have the medications prescribed by Stella's doctor—liquid morphine, liquid Ativan and the entire Urgent Care Kit which includes Tylenol in suppository form, drops for excessive saliva and other comfort measure drugs. I also have a supply of incontinent pads, a catheter kit and mouth swabs.

I am listening to a harp music CD, trying to clear my mind of the recent deaths I've attended. I must focus on Stella and her family. I realize that though I may witness deaths like this fifty times a year, this could easily be the first and only death for this particular family. The loss of a mother is earthshaking for anyone and I'm sure this will be difficult. I murmur a prayer of compassion for all concerned as I pull into the driveway.

As soon as the door opens, I'm hit with a volley of questions. "She can't be dying right now," a male voice dominates all other comments from the ten people gathered in the living room. "Please help us. I'm Joe and that's my mom, Stella." He points to a very frail woman bent over on the sofa. "Her doctor thought she was doing okay. So, how can she do this to us? We're not ready." Joe's remarks fire in rapid succession—"My sister is in Philadelphia. She has a ticket for this weekend. She promised Mom she'd be here at the end but after last night, Mom says she's done." Joe draws a sobbing breath as he finishes.

Approaching Stella, I note she is barely responsive. She is breathing very rapidly and there is panic in her eyes. I quietly introduce myself— "I'm Sharon, your nurse from hospice. Your doctor wants us to offer as much support as possible." Then I turn to Joe, "Let's get your mother into bed and make her comfortable. Then we can talk."

I again speak to Stella slowly, calmly and confidently, "You look pretty miserable here on the sofa. I think you'll feel better lying down. We'll make you more comfortable and give you a bunch of pillows to prop you up. This usually helps with breathing." Together Joe and I move her into the bedroom.

"I need to go now," Stella speaks quickly, between fast respirations. "I can't breathe. I'm very scared. Help me."

But first we have to go over the official paperwork, getting signatures from Joe to provide care for her. We do, in less than ten minutes a process that can take at least thirty, explaining the role of hospice and getting signatures. Stella's other children and immediate family members are all here, trying to help, but all asking questions. How much time does she have; should other relatives be called? I can't answer everyone for I need to evaluate and talk with Stella. Joe remains at her side, very attentive and quiet.

"Stella," I begin, "your doctor has written a prescription for liquid morphine which I have with me. It will help your breathing, slowing it down and making you more comfortable. That's what we want for you right now. Is that all right?"

"Anything that'll help," she responds between shallow breaths.

"This should make you feel better within twenty minutes," I say as I put the dropper in her mouth. "I know—it tastes terrible, but it helps."

I hear a knock at the bedroom door and two of Joe's sisters enter, wanting to know what I've done.

"You can't give her morphine—that'll just kill her," one of them screams in a hoarse whisper.

"We'll talk in the living room," I say nodding to the other room. "Stella, we're going to let you rest here for a few minutes." After assuring her I'll leave the door open so I can hear if she needs anything, I gesture for us to leave the bedroom. "Now, we'll talk."

I start very calmly, "Your mother's doctor sent us here to help her and you. Because she's struggling to breathe, I gave her a very small dose of morphine that will slow her breathing by relaxing the muscles of the diaphragm. It will also give her pain relief. Did you have a bad experience with a loved one getting morphine?" I ask looking at Pat, the daughter who had screamed.

She nods and explains that her mother-in-law died when morphine was given. "She had a terrible death. We refused to use morphine until hospice came. But as soon as she got it she died. I'm afraid that's what will happen to Mom."

"But Pat," Joe interrupts, "we need help. Let's just trust what the nurse is doing. She's the expert. Maybe your mother-in-law was ready to go and when she got relief, she let go."

It's amazing how quickly explanations can turn negativity around, I think to myself.

"Joe's right. Let's check and see if there's any change in you mother's breathing," I say looking around the room full of relatives. "Before we do, though, you should all know that her death looks very close—not because of the morphine, but because of the disease process. This is often the way lung cancer goes. People can be doing okay and then suddenly crash. Our job is to make her comfortable and help you understand what's happening," I see Joe and Pat nodding. "Regarding your sister coming in from Philadelphia, I'm not sure she has time to get here if she left today. I know this is very hard for all of you because she seemed to be doing well until last night. I have seen folks wait until the needed person arrives before they let go. Sometimes even I have been surprised by how long a person holds on. I suggest we call your sister and see if she can get an earlier flight. Many airlines try to accommodate family members for an impending death."

When Stella's children and I go back in her room, her breathing has not slowed down. Her face appears calmer, though. She has a thin smile on her lips. It's been thirty minutes, so I can give her another dose of morphine, explaining, "This amount is equal to the narcotic in one Vicodin, really a very small amount."

As I take her blood pressure and heart rate, I watch Stella, reassuring her with tone and words. "We're here for you. I'll make you as comfortable as possible, then talk some more with your kids. I'll also call your daughter in Philly and explain things to her. Now some people want to listen when I talk to their family and others don't. What would you like?"

"I want to hear," she says haltingly, between quick shallow breaths. "I know I'm dying. I just want to get it over with." She looks at each of her children. "Don't cry. I see your dad reaching out for me. I'll be all right."

Over the next half hour the ten family members and I discuss what's happening, what to expect, how we can help. Then I place the long-distance call.

"What! You've got to be kidding," Cheryl screams the words into my ear. "I just spoke to her last night. I told her I'd be there early Saturday. This can't be happening. Do you mean I can't get there in time; is that what you're saying?"

I respond as gently as possible, "Your mother is very tired and yes, it is sudden. She might make it until Saturday, but it's highly probable she won't. I will say that if you are supposed to be here, one of two things can happen: one, you will get that emergency flight, or two, your mother will wait for you. But our job right now is to make her as comfortable as possible. She's in bed and I gave her some medication to ease her breathing.

She seems better now. Know that she feels your love, with or without your presence. I know this is difficult because you want to be here holding her hand. The time of her death is in God's hands now. Your mother looks like she wants to talk to you."

I stand beside her holding the phone and hear her say, "I love you, too. I'll try, but I'm so tired. Daddy's waiting for me. I saw him just now, motioning me home. Bye, umm." She falls asleep as I take the phone.

"Yes, I'm still here. Yes, I think you should try to get that flight changed. No one knows when that last breath will be taken." I pause, listening. I give her the office number and then hand the phone to her brother.

Stella is resting comfortably, so I return to the family in the living room. I explain how Cheryl took the news. "You need to know that no one person can predict the time of death. Our job is to let go of our expectations of her. If she can wait until Cheryl comes, it'll be that way." I study the faces in the room: son and daughters, three grown grandchildren, three nieces, a nephew. "I know some people do not want their loved ones to see them take that last breath. I know of several cases where the family made a promise to be there until the end and then just when they stepped out of the room—their loved one died. I believe this is because they didn't want their dear ones to see their last breath. I think it's out of love for the family that it happens that way. Love is so very omnipresent with the dying person."

Tears mark every face, so I give hugs all around. "I'm very sorry—I know this seems sudden. But when the lung cancer is far advanced and a tumor is close to the arteries like Stella's is, occasionally a large amount of blood is coughed out. This is because the tumor has invaded the artery. This can be hard for caregivers since any amount of blood is frightening, let alone a large bleed-out. This could happen and if it does, call us immediately for reassurance."

Reading their facial expressions, I see that this is not new information. "If any of you have some dark colored towels they would be helpful, especially if she bleeds heavily." I feel like the bearer of bad tidings, but know it's better to be prepared than to leave it to chance.

"She did cough up some blood last night," Joe says, "but she made me promise not to tell anyone. She said not to worry about it. Thank you for telling us what might happen, but it's a lot to take in. Pat needs to leave for a while. Is that all right, or should we all stay?"

"I suggest that each of you take the time to be with her now, saying the things you want said. Even if she can't talk, she still hears you. Be with her, knowing this could be the last time. Your presence is so important. Sit, speak or remain silent. Then leave."

I note several family members crying as they shake their heads. Though I've made this speech many times, I know how important it is for a family to hear. I haven't spent any time with this family, so I try to condense my speech without leaving anything out. "Do the things you need to do. She's doing her heartwork, with or without speech. She'll know you love her, wherever you are, whatever you're doing." Pat smiles—faintly nods. "You might want to schedule shifts, so when one is here, the others can be called if there's a turn for the worse. As I said, none of us knows when she will pass and you'll need your strength. So take care of yourselves. I call this phase *the vigil* and it's tough. It's hard to sit when you want to be doing something for her. I can see that you all care very much for her. She's fortunate to have you here."

I sit for another hour in their kitchen, charting, making calls to arrange delivery of equipment and discussing necessary arrangements if her death occurs during the night,

Before I say goodbye, I check on Stella and let her know the family will be all right. I kiss her forehead, telling her she's done a good job. Everyone has been in to see her and only Joe remains at her bedside. He hugs me and walks me to the door. "We'll be okay. Thanks for all your hard work."

Stella dies early the next morning. Cheryl did not arrive in time but calls to thank me for letting her talk to her mother. "I knew I wouldn't make it when she said that Daddy was motioning her home. I'm just glad she was able to go without suffering."

Author's notes: Chapter 1
Death on Admission

Note 1: Hospice is a service available to all Medicare recipients and most major insurance providers. The goal is to provide end-of-life care and support to the patient and family. Requirements, admission criteria and payment to agencies are established by the government. Participating hospice agencies must follow these guidelines to qualify for reimbursement. To qualify, a doctor must determine that if the disease progresses as expected, death is likely to occur within six months. An interdisciplinary team consisting of nurses, medical social workers, bathing assistants, volunteers, chaplains, with physical and occupational therapists participates as indicated. Stella's referral came on the eve of her death. Many admissions are done in such circumstances often due to the family's or patient's resistance to hospice or to their denial. I needed to work quickly to provide the necessary education and prepare for her death.

Note 2: In Oregon, hospice personnel are not required to attend the death, but nurses will make visits if requested by the family.

Note 3: Many persons will wait for a loved one to arrive before letting go. Cheryl did not make it to be with Stella, but Cheryl did tell her that she would be alright. In an attempt to reassure the family or friends, I explain that some people do not want their loved one(s) to see them take their final breath.

Note 4: "Heartwork" is a term I use for the private time needed by the dying one before letting go can occur. For further clarification see p. 80.

"No, I don't think Joan's dying," Susanne comments. "After all, she's only 44 years old. She was fine until her family arrived."

"Suzanne and I moved up here to get me on a hospice program," Joan tries to bring me up to speed. "We tried in southern Oregon—Ashland to be accurate—but they said they couldn't see me for two months. We knew we needed help immediately, so we found an apartment here, bringing just us and our dog. Then we invited my mother and sister to come for a visit. It's been disastrous."

I had called Joan several times since her admission for end-stage lung cancer and had been told things were going okay, so a visit wasn't needed. This is not unusual since the admitting staff often answers questions and stabilizes things short term. Routine hospice visits are often refused, seen as a reminder of impending death. But now I am here on a request from Joan and Susanne. I had spoken to Joan yesterday and told her she could increase her pain medication, Oxycontin, in accord with my orders.

Joan continues her narration as soon as I sit down, "I couldn't under-stand Mom because of a stroke last year, so my sister told me how horrible Grandma's death was. She died several years ago of lung cancer just like I have. I wasn't around then and hadn't really heard all the details. Mom took care of her and I guess it was miserable. Grandma had a lot of pain." She looks at me with pleading eyes. "Please tell me it won't be like that for me. They went home yesterday, but I can't forget the look on Mom's face when she tried to talk about it."

Susanne breaks in, addressing me accusingly and states, "I think it's the medication you increased yesterday. I think it has her wired! Can't you change to a different type of medicine?"

Looking from the caregiver to my patient, I say, "Yes, I can if necessary, but first I'd like to ask this: What do you think is going on here? Really?"

Joan angrily replies: "Well, whatever it is—I am not dying." Her face is very drawn; her forehead has sunken areas at her temples. Fear is written in those lines. I sense her death is close but both women are so resistant to talking about it that I ignore my intuition.

"Are you having any pain right now?" I ask.

"No, but I'm uncomfortable. And I'm afraid," she replies. "Afraid my death will be awful!"

"I know—and fear adds to pain because your body responds by tightening up. Do you have the medication I brought yesterday?" I ask Susanne. She nods.

"Joan, I'd like to give you have some Lorazepam now. It will ease your anxiety and cut down on the intensity of the discomfort," I look over to Susanne to gauge her reaction

"Are you sure this is what she needs?" Susanne asks as she hands me the bottle. She is obviously very anxious, feeling it her sole responsibility to keep Joan comfortable. "There are so many things we want to talk about—I don't want her to be so sleepy that she can't carry on a conversation."

" I understand your concerns, but this'll help her right now. It is a small dose," I explain, "but once it takes effect she'll feel better." I put the dropper of Lorazepam under Joan's tongue. "This medication enhances the effect of the Oxycontin. I often use them together for that reason."

After a short wait, I continue, "I'm sorry your mother's visit upset you like this. But you both need to know there have been some changes in the way we treat end-of-life pain. Our job is to be aware and change drugs if one is not effective after we've reached a maximum dose. We want you to be as comfortable and as alert as possible." Then to Joan, "If this makes you drowsy, go ahead and sleep a little—I think you'll awaken with much less fear and anxiety. I promise I will do the best I can to make you peaceful, comfortable and without pain. Do you understand that?"

"Yes, I'm sorry," Susanne apologizes, looking at me.

"You've had a normal response. Sometimes medications have side effects—Lorazepam has been known to make some people more agitated. But I think this will calm her down. Here are written instructions on what to give Joan the rest of the day and into the night. Please call if it doesn't seem to be working. The dose can be increased if needed, but I want to hear from you if there's a problem."

By the time I leave, both Joan and Susanne are more at ease. Susanne has been reassured and Joan is resting. I'm certain there'll be precious words exchanged when she awakens.

The very next morning, I get a panic call. "Joan says she needs two people from hospice and she needs them right now," Susanne's voice is clearly agitated. "She wants you and the chaplain. The chaplain is already on his way. How soon can you come?"

"I'll be there in fifteen minutes." I answer calmly. "Is she having any pain now?" I ask calmly.

"No, she says she's okay with that. We got the chance to talk a lot his morning. She doesn't seem restless. I've given the meds like you told me to. Please hurry."

When a call like this comes, I know I must act quickly. I leave unfinished paperwork on my desk, asking my supervisor to take an expected call from a doctor.

"Hurry," Susanne yells as soon as I walk through the door.

As I sit on the bedside, Joan looks at me. I immediately hear her soft whisper, "Goodbye!" Joan sinks back into her pillow. Susanne and I look at her and then each other. We know she has died.

Just like that!

The chaplain calls to say he's right outside the building.

Joan wanted to make sure two persons—not just any two people, but two hospice workers—were there for her partner before she said goodbye.

Author's note: Chapter 2
Honoring Denial

Note 1: Joan has hospice coverage through her Medicare Disability insurance.

Note2: Joan's denial is very normal and needs to be handled skillfully. It is this denial which delays hospice admissions. Joan had agreed to hospice only when she knew it was absolutely necessary both for her and her partner.

Note 3: I saw Joan's sunken temples as an indication of her rapid weight loss. It indicated that death was imminent.

Too Much To Do

"What do you mean, do I have pain?" Martin responds sarcastically. "Isn't that why you're here? Didn't my doctor send you to help me with it? You guys always talk about a scale and I've yet to see a scale which could weigh my pain. Tell me that scale again." He pauses to wink at me.

"That scale helps us to measure pain and know if it's getting better or worse. The numbers range from 0—for no pain, up to 10—for the most intense pain you've ever had. With women, I usually refer to childbirth, with men discomfort from surgery or a broken bone. What's your level today?"

"I guess I'd say about an 8, but it's always here. Never goes away," he says smiling despite that fact.

Martin, a frail eighty-four-year-old, was referred by his doctor at the Veteran's Hospital to hospice for control of his pancreatic cancer pain. He's wearing three Fentanyl pain patches but continues to complain of significant discomfort.

"Would you like something done about this pain? I mean it is my job to help you with it. And like you said, this is why Dr. Tom asked hospice to come by. I can call him and suggest another type of pain control medication if what you have isn't working. I've worked with your doctor a lot and know he's very responsive to our requests to make his patients more comfortable. Would you like that?"

"No, I can handle it. Don't do anything yet. I've got too much to do around here. If you change the meds, I'll get too sleepy—can't do that. I've got to paint Janet's kitchen and then cane my raspberries. Just let me be."

That didn't go too well, I think. I remember hearing a lecture about how responsible we as hospice nurses are to keep the pain levels down but he's not about to follow my suggestions.

"Where would you like to be on that scale we just talked about?" I ask.

"I'll stay where I am, thank you," he replies.

This reminds me to clearly state his wishes in my records or risk the criticism of a national pain watchdog group monitoring the pain levels in hospice patients. I turn to his wife, Janet, who shrugs her shoulders.

"Our son is willing to do everything he wants done, but he won't let him do anything for him. He thinks he has to do it all. He didn't tell you this, so I will." She looks over at her husband of sixty-four years. "Martin's falling all the time, and he thinks it's because of the meds, so he doesn't want any more, or even to change them."

Martin lifts his shirt to show the pain patches on his chest. I remember a comment made by his doctor in the referral about Martin's driving becoming impaired due to the high narcotic dose. So now I ask if he's continuing to drive and remind them that Dr. Tom didn't want him driving across town for appointments.

"Hell, yeah," he retorts. "How else would we get to Costco? I take Janet there every week for those fabulous hot dogs. I know, my doctor said I shouldn't be driving, but I haven't fallen asleep at the wheel once, have I, Janet? I'll stop when I get dangerous."

Right, I say to myself, *just like every other man says when told to stop driving*.

Janet shakes her head, "I've told him I should drive, but he refuses to ride with me. Says I'm a poor driver. As you can see, he doesn't listen to anything I say."

"Stop talking to her," Martin interrupts in an irritated tone. "Come out back and see all the work I've done." He motions for me to follow him. "See that row of berries there? I've just cut them back and wrapped the long ones around the wires. I've got a lot more to do. Do you want to help? I'll give you some raspberries if you do."

"Where'd you get that bruiser of a black eye?" I ask Martin at my next visit.

"Oh, that's nothing. I fell off the ladder when I was painting this kitchen," he says grabbing his low back as he shows me his work. The step ladder is still in place and Janet is standing beside it.

"I told you that he's not listening. Our son said he'd do it this weekend, but he can't wait. He has to do it his way and in his time," she says, shaking her head. "I worry myself sick about him."

Seizing the opportunity for discussing pain control I ask, "Would you be willing—"

"No, it's fine, I don't need any different meds. Besides you'll probably only add another patch to my collection. Isn't that right?" He pauses for my response.

"I could use the morphine pain pump when you are ready to try something that'll work better than those patches," I offer.

"I'm not wearing that heavy thing around. I saw it once. It'll just slow me down. But I'll be more careful," he replies. "I promise."

The next morning while reading Pickles on the comic page, I find a possible explanation for Martin's unwillingness to adjust his meds. In the cartoon Earl tells his wife Opal that no, he doesn't want to take a pill for his back pain. "Pain is my way of knowing I'm still alive," he tells her. I cut the strip out to show Martin.

After Martin reads the strip, he looks at me with a twinkle and agrees, "Yup, that and the fact that I have so much to do around here. But I guess since you found me out, I could give that pump a chance, as long as it doesn't put me to sleep—can you promise me that?"

"That's one of the good things about using this pump. It won't make you fall asleep but it might relax you so you aren't as driven to get things done. It gives medication at a regular rate and when you need more relief you push a button for another small dose. It'd be like you taking extra Vicodin like you now do when you hurt, only it's more powerful," I explain. "I'll get the doctor's order and start a low dose that can be increased if the discomfort isn't eased. The machine tallies the number of times you push the button."

Martin accepts the pump but continues to report pain, while refusing to increase the strength of the medicine delivered. I attach a cord with a button for him to push when he wants an extra dose. He still complains about the pain but continues to refuses the extra doses. He remains active, continuing to fall both in the raspberries and down the steps. One day he explains that the big knot on his head is the result of tumbling into a large flower pot. "And I couldn't get out of it. I must have been quite a sight with my feet up in the air. Janet rescued me."

I chastise him after cleaning the abrasion and bandaging his arm. Then I call Dr. Tom. We have been chatting regularly regarding Martin's stubbornness and poor pain management.

When I ask him if he has any suggestions for preventing falls, the doctor laughingly responds, "No, not really. Unless you can wrap him in those packing bubbles. That way he won't hurt himself when he does fall."

Good suggestion, I think. *Especially since you are up at the VA and I'm down here in southeast Portland and you probably won't see Martin again.*

Martin and Janet are in constant conflict over her efforts to prevent him from incurring any more injuries. He says, laughingly, "She's tried to control me for sixty-four years, but she just can't do it. And she's not going to start now!"

I ask a physical therapist to make recommendations for safety and fall prevention. Martin listens to everything, agrees and then quickly returns to his colorful and dangerous style of maintaining his home.

After suffering additional pain because of several more falls, Martin finally allows me to increase the basic pump rate of the morphine delivered. His gradual decline becomes obvious to all.

I arrange a family meeting to discuss more help for Janet, but once again, stubborn Martin protests. He says, "I can't quit my riding mower, working in the yard or tending to things around my home. If I give up doing all these things, I will die. As long as I'm moving, you can't plant me. I've let Janet drive us to Costco—but we're not going there very often."

As Martin's pain becomes more manageable, he slows down but he hasn't stopped falling. He explains as I'm once more cleaning up a scraped elbow, "I guess I just forgot and took off without my walker."

Finding a big abrasion on his left arm during another visit, I hear of the night's adventure from Janet. "He refused to change places on the bed, so he'd have more room with the oxygen tanks. As he was getting up, he fell between the tank and the bed. I had to call 911 to get him up.

I'm so frustrated with him, I could wring his neck. I don't think I can take much more of this."

"Martin," I say, "don't you think it'd be a lot easier on Janet if we got a hospital bed in here? That way we could raise the head to help you breathe easier."

"Yeah, okay, but how are you going to keep him from crawling out of that bed?" Janet asks.

"We can get an alarm that will go of if he starts to get up. How about it, Martin?"

He accepts the bed and, almost as if giving up, allows me to increase the pain medication again. He continues to decline and now spends all his time in bed. He accepts a hospice aide to help him and a volunteer to help his wife. Janet is now able to get away for her own doctor's appointments and do some shopping while he sleeps or talks to his respite volunteer.

"Dad, we'll take care of Mom and your raspberries," I hear his son say to Martin, who is fading in and out of responsiveness. "We all want you to know we love you. You've done a great job all your life doing things your way."

Janet is alone, holding his hand when he breathes his last breath. I arrive just minutes after his death. I hug Janet telling her what a good job she did. Then turning, I kiss his lifeless body.

Author's notes: Chapter 2
Too Much to Do

Note 1: We, as hospice nurses, get additional training for managing pain medications. I knew I had to honor where Martin was and what his desire was for the management of his pain. He said he was satisfied with his medications because he did not want to be too sleepy to do his chores around the house. I knew I had to work with him to increase or change his drugs. This pain assessment tool is used by all medical personnel, including hospital, doctors' offices and home care nurses to provide common understanding. In hospice we report the pain level, the medication used and the number of pills needed to keep the pain controlled. Martin changed his mind and allowed me to change the medication from the patches to the pump for better control.

Note 2: There is an interdisciplinary team consisting of physical and occupational therapists, bathing assistants, medical social workers, chaplains and volunteers. Martin's frequent falls concerned me and I thought he might better heed a male therapist instead of me. It didn't make much difference. Martin loved the bathing assistant once he allowed her to help him.

Note 3: Equipment is provided by hospice and covered by Medicare and some insurance companies. The local agency has a contract with an equipment vendor.

To a Great Lady

"I've had enough of this life.
I've lived 94 years,
And there is nothing left for me.
I am never going to return to those things which gave pleasure.
I can't see,
I can't hear,
And I can't even get the words out!

"I don't want to be a burden on anyone.
I've lived my life,
And it's over!
Sure you can keep me alive for 10 more years…
But for what?
And what would be the quality of my life?

"I've had a good life:
Fishing, hiking, skiing, spending time with friends..
But no more!
Now I can't find the words to carry on a conversation-
I know what I want to say,
But it won't come out of my mouth.

"No, I'm not depressed,
I'm just complete with life.
Why is that so hard for doctors to understand.

"Please, Please,
Please let me be in control of my dying!
When can I stop my pills?
I know they are keeping me alive,
"And I do not want that any more.
Let me say good bye to my family-
No, don't tell anyone who doesn't need to know,

It's my life and I want it to be my death...
Yes, Yes, I do want to die."

What an experience,
To be brought into the confidence of this grand lady,
To witness her intention, her willingness to let go.
She expressed her desires,
Her family honored her.
She became tired, slept more,
Ate less and then
Peacefully passed thru the veil.

What a legacy for your children and grandchildren-
You knew what you wanted,
You went for it...
And I was privileged to watch.
Thank you,
Thank you for teaching me,
Even as you chose to let go.

My Last Wish

Lena's seventy-two years old. She's been struggling with pulmonary fibrosis for the last year. On my first visit, I hear the story of her much hated move to this assisted living facility along with her husband, who is also quite ill.

"You see, I lived in Gladstone in a big house and then we moved to Canby to a small apartment. It was small, but my husband Jerry and I were doing quite well. I had a place for all my things." She motions around the room, "It wasn't like this. Everything had its place. But our health got so bad our children insisted we move here." Lena's struggling not only with her own disease but also with her husband's diabetes, high blood pressure and obesity. "Now, Jerry or I can get help by just ringing the bell instead of calling the kids to come help us. They're all very busy and Jerry is getting worse. He's dependent on me but he doesn't hear me when I tell him to do something. He's at lunch now."

Looking around her apartment I imagine all the contents of a 3,000 square foot home being compressed into this 900 sq. ft. space. Compared to other apartments in this facility, this would be the biggest, yet it doesn't appear that way. There are two recliners, each with end tables. One is in the opened position with a large coffee table in front of it. It also has a large-screen television, a big sewing table, a massive dining table and chairs. Besides these there are two walkers and an oxygen concentrator with several tanks.

"I love to have my friends come over to visit," she says, interrupting my appraisal of her space. "My church friends drop by and so do my old neighbors. My quilt club meets here, too. My work friends come once a month. They'll be here tomorrow. There's a big dining room here, so that's where we meet. My great-granddaughters were here yesterday for a tea party. We sat on the floor with our tea-cups and cookies. I had fun."

At least one time per weekend, she goes out for a family visit with oxygen tanks in tow. Lena's disease requires a higher concentration of oxygen than other patients need, so when she leaves she must take at least six tanks with her. Her family is accommodating and attentive to her needs and very willing to help with the tanks.

Lena's a busy lady determined to keep productive and active. She is a seamstress and a quilter and very proud of her work. "Don't even think about telling me to give up my projects. When I finish one I'll find another one—this keeps me alive!" She finishes quickly, huffing to catch her breath.

"Thanks for coming to visit me: I like you," she says as I say goodbye.

"Mom, I promise you I'll take you to Joann's Fabric this Saturday. I know you're out of material to finish that purse," Cindy explains to Lena when she's leaving just as I'm entering. "We're going to have to do something with this mess. You've got so much stuff that the staff are starting to complain," she calls back as she starts to close the door. "Oh, I didn't see you," she's startled to see me. "Come on in. Mom really likes you. I've been telling her how we have to clean up this place. The staff says they can't clean around all this mess."

"Here, just move those things off that chair," Lena says. She offers me a folding chair she wedged between the sewing machine and her Christmas display of Kincaid lights and a circling train. The sewing machine overflows with material, thread, patterns and half-completed quilts.

"I've so much to do and Jerry seems to be adding to my worry. Yesterday, he fell in the bathroom and wanted me to help him up. I told him to use the call bell and get the staff. He wants me to do everything for him, even though he knows I can't. He even asks me to get him a glass of water—when I'm sitting down. Would you talk to him? He won't listen to me, maybe he'll listen to you." "I'm more than willing to talk with him—if he's here at my next visit," I reply.

Moving back to her chair, Lena becomes tangled in her oxygen tubing. "I wish someone would help me with this doggone thing. I'm going to choke myself on it, the way it keeps tangling," she says pulling the tubing off her head. She readjusts it after freeing it from the walker.

"I'll have to ask the staff to do more because I just don't have much energy anymore." Since this is an Assisted Care Facility, the staff can assist in personal care, bathing, vacuuming and making the beds but not other things, so I question her needs right now.

"My family came over for dinner last night, but I refused to let any of them wash the dishes. I didn't think it's right to invite people over and then ask them to wash their dishes." Knowing I can do my job while I wash them, I do so willingly.

Grateful for my help, Lena continues, "I have three daughters and four granddaughters—I want to make each of them a purse. I saw this pattern and it is so easy. And then I have three quilts I must complete," she pauses to catch her breath. Even with oxygen coming in at eight liters/minute, she is becoming winded with this long conversation. Then with renewed enthusiasm she says, "Have you seen the quilts I've made? I put them on our beds. Go in there and see Jerry's—it's a man theme" she says directing me to his bedroom. A beautiful brown and teal quilt with wildlife décor appears more professionally done than any I've seen.

"Look at the one on my bed," she says, redirecting me to her room. On her bed lies a beautiful quilt with hearts all over it. "I made one of these for each of my grandkids last Christmas. I still need to complete the ribbing on one edge before the last one's done. See here it is," she holds it up for inspection and admiration.

"What talent and love these show," I reply. I see her face beaming with pride.

"Do you know anything about computers?" she asks beseechingly. When I nod, she points toward the window where her computer, speakers and printer are squeezed into one small space. "Next time you're here maybe you can help me with mine?"

"Gosh, Lena," I reply apologetically when I see the Apple on its front, "mine's not an Apple, so I probably can't help."

As soon as I walk in several visits later, I hear, "We gotta talk. I'm so worried about my breathing. It's getting worse and I don't want to turn the oxygen meter up. I was told it would be over for me when I needed more than 10 liters/minute. So I'm trying to conserve, talk less and do less of the housework, but it doesn't seem to be working. I've got too much to do to spend my day in bed. Tell me what I'm going to do when I reach the end of the upper limits of oxygen?" As she tries to catch her breath, I see tears building up.

As I help her to her chair, I speak as calmly as possible, "Lena, let's sit for a moment. Pause, breathe in slowly, now release like you were blowing a candle out. Slowly…Now again—deep breath—pause and release." Modeling this breathing for several minutes, I start talking again slowly and compassionately, "Lena, all your decorations tell me that you are a believer in God—for just a moment I want you to close your eyes and listen to this prayer." I quote the Serenity Prayer: "God, grant me the serenity to accept the things I cannot change, the courage to change the things I can and the wisdom to know the difference. Though this is often quoted by and for alcoholics, Lena, this prayer is for you right now."

Taking her through the physiology of her breathing, I explain that eventually the lungs stiffen so that the amount of oxygen delivered will not be enough to supply the need of the body, but that is not the case right now.

"We are able get more than the limit you mentioned, if it's necessary and helpful for you. But we need to get a different machine in here. We can to do that. The equipment company is very accommodating and will work with us."

I suddenly notice her eyeliner does not run with her tears and realize they're tattooed on. The furrows of fear give way to a smile. Breathing deeply once more, Lena sighs, "That's so good to hear. I heard that comment as a death sentence. I was sure I would die as soon as the oxygen was turned up that high. And that prayer—it is so right for me. Would you write it up, so I can hang it all over my home? And would you talk to my family? They need to hear your explanation since they're the ones seeing me get all uptight and anxious. I think one of my daughters is struggling with this—we've had some issues over the years."

Finding a convenient time and space to fit the family into this apartment is difficult but proves rewarding for all concerned, including Jerry. I bring all of them up to date with Lena's process, her fears and our assistance. As a result of the meeting, I bring in a hospice aide, the chaplain and an energy worker to help provide her comfort.

Jerry's beginning to trust the staff and calls them more frequently when he needs them. The family now appears to understand more of the process. Doctors rarely get the opportunity to address an entire family, so a spokesperson generally carries information to the entire family. Here they have had the opportunity to ask questions and express feelings.

Later, Lena confides more concerns, "I'm so worried about Cindy. She and I have had so many problems over the years—with her emotions and now with my dying. She's always felt left out. I don't know how to help her."

"Lena, there are eleven words I recite for all my patients and encourage them to use them if it feels appropriate. Do you want to hear them?" I ask.

"Sure I do. You've given me so many good suggestions. Even my family said that after our conference the other night. What're those words?"

"I learned them from a hospice doctor at a conference I went to. They're useful for all of us but especially if one of us is leaving whether by death or even moving. This doctor said he's even used them for each of his children when they've left for college. They are: **Please forgive me; I forgive you; I love you;** and **Thank you**," I pause for a moment to let the words sink in.

"Wow," she says, "those are powerful words. Would you mind repeating them and please write them down. I think they'd be good for Cindy to hear. Maybe I should say them to my husband and all my kids?" She looks at me as if asking for validation.

"That, of course, is your decision, but I can't think of a better way to honor your family—if it were me," I reply.

Several visits later, Lena volunteers: "I tried to talk to Cindy, but it was very difficult for her to hear. I was able to tell some of it to Jerry, but he didn't want to hear me talk about dying at all. He says I should be more positive. I've spent time thinking, praying and there's one thing. You asked if I had unfinished business, and yes, there is one more thing I'd like to do before I die," Lena says as she looks at me with tears in her eyes. "I would like to see a man from my past. He was a beautiful friend. I want to thank him. Do you think you could help me with that?"

"Years ago, when my husband and I weren't getting along well, I fell in love with Don. He was always so easy to talk to, very different than my husband. Jerry didn't know anything about it. But we had such a great time together. We learned so much about life from each other, but he was married, and so was I." A dreamy look appears in her eyes as she tells all she gained from the time spent with Don.

"Together, we decided that it had to be over, so I've never seen him after we said good bye. I went to his daughter's funeral, but I felt awkward when his wife came up to me, so I didn't get a chance to talk to him. My daughter works with his wife who now knows about our friendship. She tells my daughter that her husband is doing well. But I never had the chance to tell him how much he meant to me. I'd like to do that before I die. Does that sound bad? It would feel so good to see him or talk to him."

"I think that's a very deep and meaningful wish. I'd encourage you to act on it, however you can. Have you thought of writing a letter, or calling him?" I ask.

"That's it! My grandson fixed my computer, so I will write one. My family knows a little about the friendship and I don't want to read it to them. You'll let me read it to you, right?" She smiles at me. She knows I will listen without judgment.

What an honor, I think. This job allows me to be present for the expression of the deep heart needs of those I walk beside in this, their last days, weeks or months of life.

Lena continues to require increasing amounts of oxygen. She has moved from 6 liters/minute to 8 and then 10 but continues to be short of breath. I add small doses of Oxycodone in order to ease that dyspnea (difficulty breathing). Since she has significant anxiety, Lorezapam is also being used on a regular basis. She's continuing to work on her projects and fortunately has been able to get the quilts done and complete most of the purses.

Several times she's run out of oxygen or had the mask fallen off during the night and she's panicked, requiring extra nursing visits but is still able to enjoy visiting with friends and family. The chaplain is very important to her as she processes feelings of fear and sadness.

"I've done it," she announces proudly one visit when she's feeling pretty good. "I've finished the letter. Can I read it to you?"

I nod my head and she proceeds to read a beautiful tribute to a cherished friend. She speaks of lessons and gifts gained from the relationship. She thanks him for being in her life when she needed his friendship.

"I gave it to my daughter to give to his wife. And he called me! It was so wonderful. He said he couldn't come to see me because he wants to remember me as I was then. He was so happy to hear from me. Thank you for encouraging me, for helping me so much. I can never repay you."

Lena smiles and hugs me. But this is followed by talk about her breathing and the continuous deterioration.

"I take some extra juice, you know which I mean, that Lor-whatever you call it, when I feel really uptight and scared," she says, looking as though she needs my approval. I agree with that, but I also increase the amount she takes and change her schedule. She fills the needle-less syringes with her medicine while I watch, and puts them in the glasses labeled Lorazepam and Oxycodone.

Over the next two weeks, the facility staff makes many calls about Lena. Their calls are regarding medication, increased breathing trouble, falling while going to the bathroom and many others, some requiring reassurance or a nurse's visit. With each change more care is required, so her daughters rotate turns staying with her to provide comfort and support.

Liquid medications are now given because she's unable to swallow pills. One evening she calls a family meeting, sure that she's dying that night. She wants everyone there. She searches the faces around the bed, mouthing I love you to each one.

When I arrive the next morning to see her, she looks up at me and smiles.

"This is what I call a practice," I tell the family. "Lena wanted you all to gather here so she could tell you she loves you and wants you all prepared."

This was the last time she acknowledges her family. Lena dies the following evening with her daughters and husband beside her.

Author's notes: Chapter 4
My Last Wish

Note 1: Lena focused on the projects she wanted to complete before she died. She had a reason to continue until she'd finished. Many folks on hospice do this, either with projects or events like the birth of the great-grandchild. They become determined to continue fighting until that event.

Note 2: Lena developed a good relationship with the equipment company since they frequented her home so often.

Note 3: I referred the chaplain and an energy worker. Both of these were very important to Lena, offering support and calming interventions. We shared our observations and suggestions in interdisciplinary meetings held regularly.

Note 4: When Lena became unable to swallow pills, I was able to get the pharmacy to provide essential medications in liquid form. As death approached we eliminated all but the medications used for comfort, breathing and pain control. Trying to give pills, food or even water when death is close can cause aspiration followed by pneumonia.

The Mystery

I sit before Death
As a conduit
Open,
Holding all emotions
Judging none,
Welcoming all.
Solid,
Grounded,
Loving,
This container is.

Resentments,
Regrets,
Sadness,
Sorrows
All blend in this vessel.
For this is Life and Death!
This is the Mystery.

It is neither judge nor doctor
Neither limiting nor curing.
It accepts all given to it,
Holding the sadness and the joys
It has a firm solid foundation,
It has no agenda,
Yet honors all where they are.

For this is the chalice of Life,
Of death,
Of the Mystery!

The Flower Man

"Wanna see what I do? Come on into my workshop," Bert says after greeting me at the apartment he shares with his wife Susanne. He turns his wheelchair, leaving me no choice but to follow him. The bedroom is an artist's workshop with shelves at wheelchair height. I note paint spills on the floor, but most of my attention goes to bright, colorful, handmade flowers.

Bert is smiling from ear to ear. I see several scars on his head and tattoos decorate his arms. His hair has been shaved. He is a big man, fully filling the wheelchair.

"I made all of these flowers. Aren't they beautiful? I make them from recycled bottles or lids. I go to the Goodwill store and visualize how I could use this or that," he proclaims proudly.

"I'm impressed," I say sincerely, knowing how unique each one is. "You are very creative."

"Yup. It helps me pass the time of day. I don't have a lot of energy for much of anything else. I give 'em away— I just gave fifteen of them to a group of church kids who came over. It makes me happy," he says smiling a big, beautiful smile.

Bert, a seventy-three year old suffering from end-stage heart disease, is delightfully stubborn. He lives with a petite wife, Susanne, who is far too sweet and very much in love with him. She too comments on his work.

"Yes, he makes lots of flowers but lots of messes too. I was down on my hands and knees cleaning up what he spilled. He was using that can of blue paint to color those." She points to a vase of blue pussy willows.

Everywhere I look I see vases full of flowers made from a variety of recycled materials. There are tulips, roses and daffodils in various stages of completion.

"What are the vases made from? Don't tell me these are juice containers," I say genuinely impressed.

"Soap bottles, pill containers, anything I can give a second life to," he says, holding up an arrangement. "This here is made from popcorn I glued on this stick and made it a pussy willow. Then I sprayed them all blue. Pretty cool, isn't it?" The other containers are sprayed green after he's made leaves and glued them on. "Look here at this set-up. I made it for someone who's lost their dog, and I want to say I'm sorry," he shows a plastic soap bottle sprayed brown with a tiny ceramic dog glued on it. A cut-out from a used card with words of sympathy is glued to a skewer and placed in the vase, much as flower shops do.

"How very creative," I comment and pick up a daffodil. "Is that what I think it is?"

"Yup, it's a top of an Elmer's glue bottle. I made the petals out of cardboard and then added the leaves to a green skewer." Six daffodils sprout from a bed of rocks in a juice container.

"You gotta see this one," Bert exclaims as he picks up an arrangement of roses with a picture of a diamond ring poking out. "I made it for someone to give to a sweetheart."

Though Susanne scolds, I see her smile. I can tell she's happy he's busy.

"Here, take this one," Bert picks up a bouquet I've been looking at. "Or would you rather have a different one? As you see, I have many to choose from. You should have seen this place before I gave some to this church group. This room was packed."

"Thank you so very much," I say, feeling honored by his gift. It is an arrangement of tulips in a cut-down quart juice container. He has gathered, folded and glued the petals in cup-like fashion. As I accept this folksy piece of art, I'm sure there will be many more gifts offered, not all in the form of a bouquet.

Susanne has been trying to take care of her sweetheart, but she's finding it more difficult because he is so "big and stubborn." Her daughter helps but has a job and a family to care for, so they are grateful for the assistance hospice can give.

"But I don't think you are going to get an aide to help him," she explains softly when he's slow getting out of his work area in his wheel-chair. "He says he only wants me to help, but it's getting very hard."

Over the next few weeks, I can see that Bert's getting weaker. Susanne reports, "It was real tough this weekend. He's so weak he had trouble getting on the toilet. That room is so tight what with the wheelchair in there."

" I almost fell between the toilet and the bathtub," Bert chimes in. "But we were able to make it. It won't happen again. I promise I'll be more careful." He appears rather embarrassed and sheepish. He's begun sleeping more and spending less time on his projects. But he continues to insist that anyone coming to his home leaves with a bouquet of home-made flowers. Every desk in my office is now decorated with this folk art.

Arriving on a sunny day, I find Bert looking a little down in the mouth. "How about I take you out on a wheelchair ride?" I ask and he quickly accepts.

"It'll do me good; maybe I'll get some ideas for my flowers," he says smiling at my offer. Pushing a two-hundred-seventy-five pound man uphill proves difficult for me, but I know Susanne at less than eighty pounds will never be able to do it. He appreciates getting outside in the sunshine.

Over the next couple of weeks he continues to have near falls getting on the toilet.

"How would you like to have that commode chair we talked about?" I ask. "We could put it in your work area. It'd be much easier for you to stand, pivot and sit down on a chair. Easier than trying to get out of the bathtub if you fell in there." At present, Bert's refused at least three times.

"That would really help," Susanne pleads with him. "I'm so afraid you will fall in that tub, and I can't lift you out. Please consider it, Bert."

"NO, no, N-O, absolutely NO," he screams. This is just what I expected. Having a commode brought in is anathema to many men. Maybe it's denial of the deterioration that many patients—not just men—display. No hospital bed, no diapers, no bathing aide, is the war cry of denial.

At my next visit, Bert is heading off to the bathroom. I follow—to find out how he's managing. "There, you see," he says when he finishes unassisted, "I'm getting better. Why don't you go back in my work area and see my new arrangement?" I'm sure he wants to divert my attention from the commode, but I obey.

"My church is bringing another group of kids over to see my flowers. They call me 'The Flower Man,' " he says as he holds the new arrangement in a one liter Coke bottle. "You understand, Sharon, I might as well give up if I'm forced to use a thing like you and Susanne are pushing. Or do you have some special interest in the potty chair business?" he chortles, laughing at his own joke. I can tell he's thinks he's convinced me to keep "that thing" out of his home.

Walking my dog that evening after work, I kick a pine cone and bend to pick it up. I think about Bert's creativity and this cone. Oh, this is perfect, I think. Maybe I can bargain with him. I put it in my pocket to take on my next visit to him. I remember how good I was at bribing my young kids to hike farther by offering M&M trail mix "when we reach that tree." It worked for them. Perhaps, I can get a commode in Bert's work area if I offer to bring some of these cones. Are bribes ethical, I wonder?

"Hey, this is great," Bert exclaims as he turns the cone over in his hands. "All I need to do is stick a skewer in them and spray them gold. They'd be beautiful in a vase, especially for Christmas with some holly leaves I could make." I can hear his wheels turning. "Can you get any more of these? I'd love to have them."

"If you give the commode a try, I'll get some more. The tree is near my home, where I walk my dog," I say, feeling proud at making a deal. "I'll bring some next visit."

"Okay, you win. I'll give it a go," he sighs, knowing he's been outfoxed.

Susanne is standing behind him. She smiles at me and then at her sweetie.

Leaving him to his flower planning, she walks me to the door. "You know, he hasn't always been this cheerful. He was quite an angry man in his youth. Many a time, he'd come home bruised, having gotten into a fight because he'd had a miserable day. That's where those scars on his head came from. He was a logger and a big strong angry one at that."

The commode is being delivered when I come later that week. I hurry into his "office" before he can wheel in, decorating the commode with a ribbon and a dozen of the highly prized cones I'd picked up. When he sees this scene, he bursts into a big belly laugh. Smiling he says, "Thanks for the cones, but I still don't want to use that thing. You drive a hard bargain."

But the wiser part of him accepts the commode and he thanks me for it the next time I see him.

Bert is now more willing to receive other offers of assistance including a hospital bed, a hospice aide and even medication to help him with his shortness of breath. I think he must be more trusting now.

"There are parts of my life that I am not proud of," he opens up one day and starts talking about his past. "I would clobber the first person who crossed my path some days. But, you know, I think I have made up for that by making these flowers and giving them away. I must be keeping the devil off my tail. Wait a minute," he pauses and smiles before continuing, "This is beginning to sound like a confession from a dying man. That's not me." He winks and changes the subject. Then he shows me the wonderful flowers he's made using the cones. I feel warm inside.

As his shortness of breath increases, Susanne gives him several small doses of morphine during the day, squirting it under his tongue. Bert only makes it to his work area for short periods, but he still insists that anyone who comes to see him leaves with a bouquet of "love" as he calls it.

Eventually Bert is transferred to an inpatient hospice facility as Susanne is no longer able to care for him. He is diabetic, unable to eat and has increasing pain and shortness of breath. She's unable to turn him or move him up in the hospital bed.

"Since I can't get there until tonight when my daughter comes home," Susanne calls the day after he's transferred, "could you go and tell him I'll be okay and that I said it's all right for him to go be with Jesus. That's just in case we don't make it in time. There's a lot of traffic going across town. I know he's failing quickly." I hear sobbing.

Bert doesn't respond at first when I visit him at the hospice facility, but as I talk to him, he rouses at the sound of my voice. He starts to chuckle and then wheezes.

"Susanne says to tell you she's all right. She's going to miss you, but she wants you to know that it's okay for you to go home to be with Jesus now." Susanne's message is received with a smile, but by the time she and her daughter arrive he's not responding .

Since hearing is the last sense to go in the dying process, hospice staff encourages families to share words of comfort with their loved one. A nurse there tells me later that Susanne kissed and told Bert she'd be alright.

Bert dies the next day but appears to me in a dream that night. He stands at the foot of my bed, laughing his big belly laugh as he pulls my great toe.

Author's notes: Chapter 5
The Flower Man

Note 1: With his doctor's approval I got liquid morphine for Bert's shortness of breath. It relaxed the diaphragm and eased his difficulty breathing. I started with a very small dose given in a syringe without a needle and placed under the tongue for more rapid absorption. Susanne was hesitant at first to give it to him but soon learned its value. Many people resist the use of morphine and require explanation.

Note 2: I had developed a good relationship with the equipment company so I was able to arrange for a date of delivery that coordinated with my next visit. This company also picks up the equipment when it is refused or when death occurs. Bert didn't know I had scheduled the delivery.

Note 3: I had Bert transferred to an inpatient hospice facility since Susanne was no longer able to provide the necessary care, and I knew he was very close to death. Inpatient facilities vary in terms of admission criteria.

Breaking the Code

"Why does he keep saying, 'I want to go home?' " Lisa asks. "He's lived here for forty years; my sister and I were born here. But he keeps asking for his shoes, saying either he has to go home or go upstairs. This is the home he built in the seventies right after he and Mom were married; he knows there's no upstairs. I don't understand," she says with tears in her eyes.

David is only sixty with a wife and two daughters living in a beautiful, spacious home. The pain from his pancreatic cancer has been difficult to control. His face appears drawn, punctuating his tremendous weight loss. Because of a recent hospitalization, he's developed a pressure sore on his heel which requires daily bandage changes.

I listen as his daughters, Lisa and Kelley and wife Connie look expectantly at me as if I had all the answers. Connie and I have just moved him from his beautifully decorated bedroom into a hospital bed situated in the living room, and I've given him a dose of pain medication.

"We can't understand why he doesn't want to eat and live longer with us," Connie says. "We've done everything we can for him. Lisa's practically given up her family to be here and help me. Kelley was with him when he told his doctor that he wanted to fight this and get better—why isn't he?"

Once David's pain is relieved, we sit near his bedside, and I softly explain what I have gained from so many people close to death. "People who are reaching their own readiness often know their families have difficulty with letting go or understanding their process. Many patients feel it is giving up or that their families will think so. They aren't cowards and would never 'give up the fight,' but at some point they come to a place where the disease takes control and they give in to the process of dying. I think David is at this place—he is using what I call 'code' talk because he is not sure you're ready to let him go. I see this often. The 'death' word can be very harsh. Letting go—see how we can use some words that are softer than saying 'death'? I think he is referring to home and upstairs as heaven. Many people talk about going upstairs or home. He probably feels he needs his shoes to leave this world. I believe David is trying to let you all know how he's feeling about death. This phase is part of the process and it takes as long as it takes. Does this make sense?"

One by one I hear a sniffle and see tears. "But I don't like it!" Connie wipes her eyes. "It seems like it was just yesterday that he was getting into our bed with my help. It was only three weeks ago when he insisted he was getting better. So why isn't he eating anything? We made his favorite pudding, got him ice cream that he loves but he doesn't want any. Are you sure this is what he is saying? I don't want to let him go unless I know for sure that's what he wants."

"Remember what I told you and David the first day I saw you? I told him that he had his hands on the steering wheel and that we are all are just traveling along with him as co-pilots. But I also said the disease has its foot on the gas pedal, and it will determine the speed we all travel," I reply, though I know I haven't answered her questions. "This disease is going fast right now."

Connie says that, yes, indeed she remembers but wondered at the time what it actually meant: "David had always been in control and I thought he would remain that way. Are you saying that we should let him starve?"

As she speaks, David awakens, yelling: "Bring me my shoes; I've got to get out of here!"

I walk over, taking his hand in mine, "It's okay, you are free to go. You don't need your shoes. You are right just as you are."

Connie, Lisa and Kelley join me. They look at their father and husband with tears in their eyes: "It's all right, Daddy, we're here and we'll stay here." Connie sobs, "David, it's okay, we're going to be all fine, but we'll miss you." Leaning down, she kisses his cheek.

Addressing Connie's question, I say, "David, you can eat if you want and when you want. If you don't want to eat, your family understands. There may come a time and it may already be here, that you don't want to eat or can't swallow well. Then we'll use these sponges on a stick." I hold up a swab for all to see. "This way, you can suck the water out of it and keep your mouth from drying out. Your family can use it to moisten your lips and mouth when you are no longer able to do that," I demonstrate its use by placing it in a glass of water and then gently dabbing his lips.

This family has tried so hard, pleading with him to eat and take crushed pills. They have held him up between them to exercise him, 'so he wouldn't lose his strength.' Now, they are present for him, stroking his hair and holding his hands. He temporarily calms at their touch and soft voices.

But after my explanation, David becomes more agitated. His need to stay in control is very obvious. Things aren't the way he intends, and he is making his discontent known to all. His family remains very present, reassuring and comforting yet worried that he is in distress—both emotionally and physically. After the use of the relaxant Ativan proves ineffective, I consult with his doctor. I start a subcutaneous (small gauge needle secured under the skin) injection. This is for a relaxant to be given continuously. Now, his family has some quiet time with him.

David can now tell them of his love for them, and he thanks them for being there. They sit with him, comforting as needed.

Several days later I am called back to comfort the family as David takes his final breaths. A soft Christmas carol plays in the background. David appears comfortable but is reaching up toward the ceiling.

"That is very normal," I say, responding to their questions. "I often think there is someone on the other side greeting them with open arms. I've had people identify family members who've died. One woman called out to her dad with her arms extended and then wrapped them in a hugging gesture. One woman said she saw Jesus coming toward her in a boat."

Lisa cries and smiles at the same time: "That makes sense. Dad's been doing that all day. I thought something was wrong. Is this another of those *code* things you talked about?"

"Yes, it is."

David's breathing slows and then stops. He takes a final gasp as his family holds his hands.

Author's notes: Chapter 6
Breaking the Code

Note 1: Hospice nurses are trained to provide wound care and make the visits necessary to either heal the wound or teach the family how to handle them. I made visits every other day until the heel wound was gone.

Note 2: David used words his family would accept. When I clarified them, he acknowledged their accuracy, so I relayed that to his family. This is common in my practice. I've found many unwilling to say they are ready to die, but they say that they are in their own way—for example saying that they need to "get home" or "go upstairs." I believe that David knew his family wanted him to keep fighting, but he was too tired to do so.

Note 3: Hospice medical directors are specially trained to offer suggestions regarding effective drugs. Many family doctors depend on the hospice doctor and the nurse to manage symptoms, since while on hospice, the patient is often not able to see their family doctor. Communications are continued with the family doctor.

Note 4: Injectable medications are not routinely used in the home setting unless there is a central intravenous line through which pain medications can be administered. This is case specific but includes tube feedings and rehydration liquids. David's doctor was the hospice director, so he was able to facilitate providing David's anti-anxiety drugs.

PART TWO

Family Dynamics

"Can you come quickly? This is Ray. I'm Steven's son. You saw us yesterday." The panicky voice continues, "My dad is climbing out of bed. He's very confused, agitated and determined to get up. I'm afraid he'll fall." Ray takes a deep breath before answering my question, "No, we don't have any rails on the bed. Please come as soon as you can."

"I'll come right away but listen to me right now. Do you have the liquid medication I left yesterday?" I ask, only to hear a pause. "It has the label Lorazepam on it. Remember, we talked about giving it to him if he needed it. Have you given any to him? It sounds like he needs it now."

"Yes, it's here. I don't think I can give him any, though. My sisters think it'll kill him; they'll blame me if he dies before they get here. They made me promise to hold all medication. Just hurry, please," Ray says with the urgency in his voice increasing."

"I'll be there in twenty minutes. Even though your sisters don't want him medicated, I want you to give a very small dose, just to the first line on the dropper. It won't hurt him. It probably won't calm him down much, but it's important to give it now just to get a little in him to begin the calming effect. Put it under his tongue like I showed you. I'll talk to your sisters later."

Fifteen minutes later, I find Ray trying to keep his father in the bed by talking to him and telling him he's too weak to walk. The small dose of Lorazepam he did administer has had little effect.

"I'd swear he's just eaten a steak instead of being a man who hasn't eaten in over 10 days," Ray exclaims as his father struggles to get up by pulling on his arms.

"Steven, what's going on?" I ask looking into his fear-stricken eyes. "Do you need something? Are you in pain?"

"I hurt all over and I gotta pee, NOW!" he yells. When I offer him the urinal, he knocks it out of my hands. "I gotta stand to pee."

"Here's something for your pain," I say reaching for the bottle of liquid morphine. "Take this and I'll get you up to use the urinal. Open your mouth for this bitter medicine." Steven makes a face but swallows the dose followed by a chaser of orange juice. It would have been better to have him hold it under his tongue but this is no time to quibble.

Together Ray and I are able to stand Steven up. But when he is unable to urinate, we gently lay him back down.

"Quite frequently the need to urinate will make a person very restless. How long has it been since he used the urinal?" I feel no moisture on the bed.

"I haven't changed his pad in over 24 hours," Ray responds. "Is this why he's so flipped out?"

"Could be," I say. "Let me catheterize him and see if that does it. But it could be fear or pain. Since we've just medicated him that should soon help. Are your sisters on their way here? I'd like to talk to them about his condition."

"Yes, I've called. They're on their way."

It is quite a challenge to catheterize an agitated man, but I succeed and a large amount of urine flows into the bedside bag. But Steven is still restless, agitated and confused when his girls arrive. Both women appear frightened and anxious.

"What do you think is happening to your father?" I ask after letting them express their concerns, especially about giving him medication.

"You understand that your dad is very close to death, don't you?" I ask them as they attempt to calm their father down. "I've given him some pain medicine since he complained of pain. Earlier I told Ray to give him some Lorezapam to calm him down. I want you to know that his dying is not because of the medications but because lung cancer is causing his systems to shut down. Medications help to make him more comfortable and get some rest. Ray says your dad hasn't slept for several nights. Is that right, Ray?" I turn to him for verification and he nods.

"Have any of you ever tried to calm a two year-old when she is so exhausted that she just cries and cries and cries?" I ask. Everyone nods, appearing unsure of the direction I'm going.

"Do you remember how you placed your hand on her back and held it there? Remember how she protested and wiggled, attempting to free herself so she could get up and run around again?" I ask. "Well this is a little like that. Your father could be frightened or in pain and we need to be like that wise parent or grandparent who offers love and calmness. His pain and fear need to be treated with medication so we can give him some peace."

"Will he wake up after he goes to sleep?" Ray asks appearing frightened and accepting.

"That depends on how much we give him and whether he is ready to let go. Many people have work to do inside their hearts and that can continue even with the medication. I've seen folks who let go immediately and others who hold on for a while, waking up and talking —until it's their time to go. You can talk to him and he'll be able to hear you since hearing is the last function to leave. Does this make sense to you?" No one answers so I continue. "Many people at the very end of life complain of pain all over—even the slightest touch may cause them to cry out in distress. That's what I see here with Steven. So, with your permission, I'd like to make him comfortable and less frightened. Is this okay?" For a brief moment I look at each of them, waiting for acknowledgment and permission.

With tears in their eyes, they nod, caressing his hands as if rubbing in their love. Ray says with a hint of a smile, "You're the expert on death here. I'm sure you've been present for many families that go through this."

So with their permission, I give Steven moderate doses of Lorazepam and morphine. After twenty minutes, he is calm and sleeping soundly. The family has arranged for shifts during the night. They are instructed in mouth care and I tell them to call if they have any concerns.

As I listen to the next day's report of deaths occurring during the night and hear his name, I say a little prayer for Steven and his family.

Ray answers when I call with condolences, "My sisters said he was calm all night. They were all right with him not talking both accepting of him not talking since they were able to tell him how much they loved him—he squeezed their hands when they told him how much they will miss him. They called me at four A.M. when his breathing changed, so we were all here when he took his last breath. Thank you for all you did to make his death peaceful."

Author's notes: Chapter 7
Calming the Anxiety

Note 1: When Steven was admitted, orders were obtained for managing symptoms of anxiety, pain and comfort. I had taken the urgent care kit (specific medications commonly used) from the pharmacy and instructed his son Ray in their use. These drugs are provided in the case of an urgent need in the middle of the night when no pharmacies are open.

Note 2: Hospice nurses are on call 24/7 so they can be available either by phone or in person for those emergencies. I, as Steven's primary nurse, happened to be on duty to answer Ray's panicked call, so I immediately went to assist.

Note 3: Steven's inability to urinate caused most of his anxiousness. Difficulty urinating is a common factor in agitation at the end of life.

Miriam's grown son John greets me at the door with a toothless grin that stretches from ear to ear. I am immediately aware that he is mentally challenged. "We wondered who they were gonna send out for Momma," he says and leads me on a little path through magazines, newspapers, groceries and books to Miriam's bedroom. My first thoughts are that I'm in for a surprise and a challenge. I've entered a hoarder's paradise with the stacks of boxes in general disarray. Empty pill bottles lie all around the room, and I hear Miriam crying out with pain. She has end-stage lung cancer.

"No, Momma, it's not time for your pain medication," John yells at the pale, emaciated woman in the bed. "You'll have to wait another hour. Can you just talk to this lady here?"

Miriam looks up at me, her tiny, childlike face contorted in the grimace of pain. "Can you help me? You're from the doctor's office, right? They tell me they'd send someone to help me. That guy said he couldn't do anything more for me, so he sent me home to die. I'm really hurting right now."

"I can see that and yes, I'm sent here by your doctor to help you manage the pain. Can I see the pills he's given you, please," I ask her, but turn to John for a response.

"Don't ask me, I don't have anything to do with that. My sister Sally gives them to her, but she told me when she left for the store that she couldn't have any more until 1:00," he answers defensively. But he goes out and returns with the bottle. "She gave her one of these and told me she couldn't have any more."

The directions clearly read to take one or two every hour if needed. Doctors are generally very liberal for pain control for cancer patients, especially those referred on to hospice.

"Here, Miriam," I say handing her one of the breakthrough pills—so called because they are fairly quick-acting and are to be used between the scheduled heavy-duty pain pills.

John frowns, "My sister's gonna be mad at you. She gets that way with me when I don't do what she says. Sometimes she's real mean."

I look up and smile, "That's all right, John. She can get mad at me. I don't want your mother in pain." As I look at him, he's standing there, his red hair long and unruly, his bibbed overalls tucked into his boots. Grass clippings are falling onto the floor but are barely noticeable among the litter.

Within minutes Miriam tells me, "The pain's getting better. I'm glad you came when you did. It was getting unbearable. What's your name, anyway? I knew you were the nurse. You called this morn and said you'd be out here. John, you go on out there now and finish that lawn. You were supposed to already have it done. Here," she says to me as she scoots over and pats the bed beside her, "sit."

"How do you get around in here?" I ask, noting that the path between the tall stacks of newspapers isn't big enough for a walker, let alone a wheelchair.

"Oh, I manage fine. I leave the walker over there and then hang on to the bed and dresser to get to it," she explains. "It's real hard, getting the walker down those two steps leading into the living room or the bathroom. Sally has to help me down there," she pauses, patting the bed again. "Come on up, Pepper, meet Sharon. She'll be coming here to see us," she says affectionately. Up jumps a tiny dog with a big bark. He's a cute little black and white hairless Chihuahua. They exchange nose kisses.

Sally greets me as she comes through the door. "So, how's my mom doing? That damn doctor told her she was dying, and he couldn't do anything for her. Is she dying? Please don't tell me that." Sally towers over me—she's about five foot eleven and weighs close to three hundred pounds. Her hair is unkempt, fingernails dirty, but real concern is written all over her face.

"Let's go into the living room," Miriam says as she gets out of bed. Sally holds out her hand to steady her mother and guides her over to the walker and then down to the living room. "Now," Miriam says as she settles on the sofa, "now let's talk."

"Why in God's name would a doctor say that to anybody, let alone my mother? You can see for yourself how much weight she's lost since she finished those radiation treatments. It was tough getting her out for those; she nearly fell lots of times. And now she can't eat because of the radiation. I don't understand. Why would he have had her continue that if it wasn't going to work?" She asks.

"Ladies," I say gently. " I don't know why doctors do what they do, but I do know they are interested in you getting better. They thought the treatments might work, but sometimes they're very hard on the body. Did you talk about this in the beginning?"

"Yes." Sally answers for her mom. "Yes, we talked about it, but we didn't know this is the way she would now be when it was over. Didn't they know she wouldn't be able to eat? How am I supposed to get her to eat?"

"Miriam's lung cancer did not respond to any of the interventions the way the doctors thought she would," I explain. "It's the cancer that is causing the decline. But the treatments were tough, weren't they, Miriam?" I ask gently.

"Yes and I never want to go back to the hospital," she says emphatically. "I just don't want to be in pain anymore."

"That's what hospice is all about," I respond. "We'll get the right pills or liquids here to keep you comfortable. Does this sound okay? By the way, Sally, I gave your mom another of her breakthrough pills before you got here. She seems better now. I want you give her two at a time until I get some liquid pain med in here. Is that all right with you?"

Sally nods, appearing grateful that someone is helping to manage her mother's pain. I think Sally didn't understood the directions, or Miriam refused to take two at a time. There are many reasons patients don't want the full suggested dose. They could be afraid they'll run out or be constipated. Too, they might think they'll look better to their family if they only take one pill at a time.

I deliver liquid pain medication at my next visit several days later and immediately hear more of Sally's concerns. "Mom nearly fell twice last night. She insists on getting to the bathroom on her own. Is there anything we can do?" She asks.

"Pain meds can cause unsteadiness, especially for a fragile person. It's going to be important for her not to go to the bathroom by herself. I could get a commode, but I don't see where we could put it," I say.

Sally is eager to make room for the commode, and we begin moving some of the stacked items, clothes, boxes and dog food around. That done, I make a call for the commode.

"Miriam, do you think the pain's better now?" I ask.

"Yes," she nods, "but I can't swallow those damn pills. I hope this stuff you brought will work better."

"We'll need to be very careful with the amount you use. You're getting weaker, and it's more difficult to get around. Sally, I want to make sure you start her with the smallest dose and repeat the same dose if it doesn't help the pain," I say, holding the dropper and pointing to the first line. "I will have you increase this the next time I see you if you are needing to give it to her more often. So, please write down the times you give it. That'll help me as I adjust the dose."

As I'm getting ready to leave, I start to hug Miriam but Sally quickly says: "You better watch out. Pepper is pretty protective of Mom." By then the hugs over and I turn to hug Sally. As I do so, this little dog grabs my butt and hangs on. I yelp in surprise as he sinks those sharp little teeth into my pants and skin.

John, who's been listening from the other side of the room, starts laughing uncontrollably. "Wow, Pepper really like nurses, doesn't he?"

I am screaming now like I was in a Laurel and Hardy movie with this dog hanging on my butt. She and Sally are apologetic, but John continues laughing and pointing at me until the dog lets go and runs to Miriam.

I leave, rubbing my buttocks, dismayed and in pain. I call my supervisor and then stop at Starbucks where I use the bathroom mirror to see if my skin is punctured. I'll need an ER visit if it is. Fortunately there's no blood, only teeth marks. I've used this coffee shop often, but never for this.

The next day, I'm told that Miriam has fallen and has been taken by ambulance to the hospital. The hospice night nurse had determined an ambulance was needed to get her evaluated for a hip fracture.

When I arrive at the hospital, I find that Miriam does have a fractured hip and is heavily sedated with pain medication. Sally and I participate in a discussion regarding surgery for repair, and it's decided not to operate considering the cancer and metastasis. Miriam's pain will be managed by an intravenous drip of morphine. The next day the family is there asking for more explanation when I arrive.

Miriam appears comfortable but isn't responding due to the massive doses of pain meds necessary to make her pain-free.

John smiles when he sees me and turns to his mother, "Mom, wake up. It's Sharon. You know her. She's the one Pepper bit," he laughs as he says it.

Miriam opens her eyes, smiles and squeezes my hand and then drifts back to sleep.

John tells the hospital nurse adjusting her pillows, "Yeah, my dog Pepper really likes eating nurses." He then asks how the bite is doing.

I pull up a chair and hold Miriam's hand, while reassuring John and Sally that she will be drifting in and out of consciousness. They're glad that she's comfortable but I think they both know it is only a matter of days before their mother dies.

Hospitals are generally very accommodating to hospice families and the staff is very sweet with Miriam's children. They are encouraged to stay as long as they like. Some families prefer their loved one be with professionals. There's worry in many home settings as to whether the care they give is good enough or if they are doing as much as professionals might do. I believe this is the case here. I show them how to dab a moist toothette on her dry lips. I reinforce the hospital nurse's comment about not waking her to ask questions. They sit quietly for a while and then leave. As they are leaving they state that they will not be able to make it to the hospital again due to Sally's fear of traffic.

Miriam dies several hours later, comfortable and out of pain.

Author's notes: Chapter 8
Pepper Loves Nurses

Note 1: When admitted to hospice, Miriam and her family were asked to identify her wishes on a paper which was then sent to the physician for signing. This is the *Physician Order for Life-Sustaining Treatment* (POLST), and it becomes an order for emergency personnel when they come to the home. The family is taught to take it with them if they need to go to the hospital.

Note 2: Miriam is admitted to a hospital while on hospice because of her fracture from a fall. Hospice has nurses on call twenty-four hours/day to handle most concerns. They make the call for an ambulance transfer when that is needed. It is a myth that no one goes to the hospital while on hospice.

Note 3: Hospice nurses visit their clients daily while in the hospital to coordinate care with the hospital.

Questions and Promises

"When will he die?"

"I have plans"

"I need to go to work"

"I must to go on this trip"

"Can you promise me
He'll be here when I return?"

"How can I be present for him
When I must take care of myself?"

"Can he hold on for two more weeks?
Then I can sit here and hold his hand"

"Please, tell me I can do this one thing."

Life flows in its own rhythm,
No one tells the bulb when to sprout.
The seasons are under no one's orders
Once engaged in the birth canal,
It's hard to keep the baby from crowning.
Once engaged in the death canal,
It's impossible to predict or control that last breath.
Like Life, Death follows its own schedule.

So,

I say,

Go to work,

Do what must be done.

Your hearts are connected,

Those who are supposed to be here,

Will be here,

Regardless of plans made,

Or promises given,

Death follows no one's agenda.

ANTIBIOTICS OR NOT

"Yes, you can help—you can explain why a doctor told me to get these antibiotics down my wife when she's not eating or drinking anything," Merwyn, Gloria's husband says. Gloria lies on the bed not responding to anything or anybody. She has just been released from the hospital and has recurring diarrhea. She was operated on for colon cancer two months ago with the promise that she'd be able to do her annual snow-birding, something which she and Merwyn have done with two other couples for the last eighteen years. He'd been planning the trip when her diarrhea returned with a vengeance. She now appears frail, near death.

"I don't understand why a doctor would tell us that giving my wife food won't keep her from dying and then orders antibiotics and tells me I must give them to her. She went to the hospital two months ago and was diagnosed with cancer. Now she's not even talking to me—look at her lying there in that bed. We've cleaned her up three times already this morning and I can tell she's had another accident now. Will you help me?" Merwyn asks with tears in his eyes. "My daughter has been kind enough to stay here with me and support her mom. She's just left to get a nap."

I help him bathe and turn his wife, using provided pads to help avoid frequent sheet changes. Merwyn's tenderness is obvious as he washes her. When she appears comfortable, I sit and talk with him. "I don't know why pills were prescribed when Gloria can't swallow. Sometimes physicians are unable to tell folks there's nothing more to be done. They subscribe to the theory that as physicians, they are a failure if they're unable to help. Your doctor also knew how important it was for you to do all you could to help her. This diarrhea is caused by a certain bug that usually responds to antibiotics; however, considering Gloria's condition, I doubt it will help."

When I come back the next day her daughter Michele is sitting at Gloria's bedside holding her hand. Merwyn is in the kitchen trying to crush the large pill using a ball-peen hammer. "I think I might have gotten one bite in her mouth this morning. I'm going to mix this one with some applesauce Gloria made from our own apples. But she closes her mouth when I offer it to her—and she holds her lips tight together. Is she trying to tell me to stop forcing her to eat or take the pill?" he asks as he scrapes the pill-powder off the breadboard.

"Possibly," I answer, "I think she is doing her best to thank you for your efforts but also to say she's ready to let go. Many folks are ready before the family is able to say good-bye. Just remember that you did as much as you possibly could. I tell families to do whatever they need to so that three months down the road they're won't hold themselves guilty for not doing enough to keep their loved one alive. The doctor knows how important it is for you to do everything possible for Gloria. And you've done that." I pause to read his expression.

"Are you saying she's dying right now?" Merwyn speaks as their daughter looks over at me. She has a knowing look even while tears flow down her cheeks.

I gently draw him to his wife's side. When he and Michele each touch her hands, I say, "Yes, I believe her death is very close. She's no longer squeezing your hands like she did. She's unable to swallow her saliva and it's been several days since she ate anything. I don't think it's safe to continue giving her any medicine. If she breathes while it is in her mouth, it could end up in her lungs and cause pneumonia. Here I'd like you to use these swabs," I show them a cardboard stick with a small sponge on the end of it, " These are to give her moisture and to wipe away the saliva. When you place this in her mouth, she can safely suck on it. She'll get the fluids she wants, and it won't go down the wrong pipe into the lungs. Does this make sense?" They both nod.

"The next phase is when she won't open her mouth at all. You can use lip balm on her dry lips. She may moan at any movement even when you're just touching her but mostly when she's turned. There is often a strange gurgling sound which sometimes frightens folks—they think their loved one is suffering when they hear it. But it's normal. I describe it as what we experience when we're sucking a milkshake through a straw. At the end of the shake, there's a sort slurping. She's not suffering, just breathing through the fluid in her mouth."

"How long will it be before she stops breathing?" Merwyn asks. "What will we do when that noise starts? I'll be so frightened I'll want to call you. What about you, Michele?"

Michele looks up and says, "We'll be OK, Daddy." Then to me, "Are there things we should do when that happens?"

"There's a couple of things you can do," I reply. You can turn her on her side and allow her saliva to drain naturally, or you can give her that small dose of liquid morphine I showed you earlier. It can be given every four hours if needed. It'll help relax her breathing muscle, the diaphragm so she can breathe easier. That would also help with any pain she could experience. Have you noticed any groaning when you move her?"

"We stop turning her when she moans. We wait a while and then finish the job," Michele says.

"In that case, it would be wise to give that dose about twenty minutes before you turn her," I explain. "Then she will be without pain when you need to clean her up and turn her. If the first dose doesn't seem to help ease her, you may repeat it and then the next time give her a larger dose—up to the second line on the dropper. Do you understand how to increase the morphine if necessary?"

"Yes," Michele nods, "but do you think she could die tonight?"

"Yes." I look first at Merwyn and then Michele. "She could. If either of you have any questions, feel free to call this hospice number." I point to the office number on the refrigerator. " If she dies and you would like a visit, our night nurse will come."

"What will you do if we ask for a visit? Merwyn asks. "Don't you need to pronounce her dead—or can I do that?"

"No, unlike some states, Oregon doesn't require someone to pro-nounce death when hospice is involved. It is regarded as an expected death. When I come out after a death, I can help bathe and dress her and get her ready for the mortuary pickup. You just need to make one call—to hospice—and we'll make the necessary calls to the doctor and the mortuary. I could also place a request in for a harpist to come and play music for Gloria, if you'd like. Harp music is very soothing, often referred to as transition music. We use a group called 'Sacred Flight'—it'd be at no cost to you. Would you like that?" I ask.

"That would be lovely," both Merwyn and Michele say in unison. Merwyn adds, "She loved to play the harp CD we have. I didn't think much of it. But I think I could find it and play it for her now."

Gloria is comfortable, with no moaning, when I help turn her after the medication. Sacred Flight is on the way. I give my final instructions. I do not know that I'll be called back before the day is over.

The harpist calls two hours later to say that Gloria took her last breath during the music session. I arrive in time to help Michele bathe her dear mother with special bath oil and dress her for her final journey.

A week later I receive a beautiful card in broad-stroked calligraphy:

My heart aches to tell you how much hospice meant to us. You made a difficult task so much easier for me and my father. Thank you so very much.

Michele and Merwyn

Author's notes: Chapter 9
Antibiotics or Not

Note 1: Gloria was given antibiotics as a treatment of last resort for persistent diarrhea. Antibiotics are used while on hospice if they provide comfort.

Note 2: I brought in the harp player because I could see she Gloria was very close to dying. I have found this adjunctive therapy very soothing and calming for patient and family. Many agencies familiar with thanatology programs provide musicians to offer harp and other soothing music for end-of-life support. But they can be beneficial throughout the hospice experience.

Note 3: Physicians find conversation regarding end-of-life care difficult as in Gloria's situation. The doctor's emphases have always been on saving lives, so it is tough for them to talk about death without feeling they have failed in some way. Hospice is often brought in because we can talk more easily about it.

Note 4: Gloria's refusal of proffered food was a signal for her family that it was no longer needed. Not eating is not painful for the loved one, though it is hard to watch. Many think they are starving the loved one. What is needed now is not physical food but love and comfort.

WHERE ARE THE SIGNS?

"I want to make sure that no one makes me live longer than I am supposed to. I don't want more promises or things given to me. I want my dying to be as natural as possible," are the first words Melanie says to me. She is being admitted for ovarian cancer and has already been through the interventions. She was recently told that nothing else could help.

Melanie's daughter, Loretta, sits beside her and half-smiles at me as she speaks: "Mom has been getting intravenous fluids through her port and she has told me that she wants no more of that. My sister says that's not the way it will be—but I want Mom to have her final say." The port is a small dime-sized device under the skin of the upper chest, connecting to a vein which is used to give the chemotherapy and later to hydrate if fluids can't be swallowed or kept down. I have been told of the family conflict over this.

A light shines from Melanie's eyes and I know immediately that we are going to be friends. She is wearing a pink turtleneck sweater and sweatpants. She has no hair but the biggest smile I've seen in a while.

"You are the queen—that's what all my clients on hospice are—and you get to do what you want when you want," I tell her. "Sometimes I think I should carry a tiara with me for this first visit—it's important for you to know how I feel from the get-go. I say if a person on hospice doesn't want to eat, she shouldn't have to and if she wants to eat ice cream all the time, then that's what she should do."

Our eyes meet with that knowing look. "Thank you." Melanie replies. "But Beth won't agree. She tells Loretta I must eat well every day to keep my strength up," She hastily throws a look at her daughter, Loretta.

Perhaps there's more here that meets the eye or ear, I think.

Loretta explains that her sister Beth is at odds with the family for bringing hospice in and also with the financial situation between them. The social worker will have more to work on with this issue than I do. I offer to talk to Beth regarding any changes in her mom's physical symptoms, but the social worker will need to address financial matters.

Melanie quickly diverts the conversation, pointing to the feeders out the window and asking if I like hummingbirds. "This recliner is where I can sit and watch them come and visit me." Melanie takes me outside, showing me all her flowers, ending at the southwest corner of her yard. She points to a shady spot, "This is where I want to build an altar for myself. I want Loretta to have a place to come and talk to me. I'm going to plant a Peace Rose here."

"You obviously love to garden, don't you?" I say as I admire her well-manicured yard.

Over the next few months as summer turns to fall, I comment on the blooms on a tree next to her window. She replies: "I had that Chinese dogwood planted there so I'd have flowers in the late fall—pretty isn't it? Life around me including me—is kinda shutting down—all except this dogwood." Melanie is declining, but she continues to get outside daily, now with the help of a cane. The Peace Rose has been planted with some stones surrounding it.

She seems to accept the toll the cancer is taking and now appreciates having a hospital bed by her living room window. "From here, I can see all the beautiful birds coming to my feeder. Look, there's a chickadee—get away you pesky starlings!"

The social worker has connected with Beth in an attempt to help her understand how this family can be healed or at least understand Melanie's wishes. Melanie has promised her house to Loretta since Beth has a large home for her family on the other side of town. Beth is also disputing her mother's decision to let the process happen naturally without further measures. Her anger has increased over Loretta's recent decision to honor their mother's choices and bring hospice in.

Over the summer, the social worker's phone calls and visits seem to improve the situation. Beth now agrees with her mother's decision to stop fighting the disease. She says that as along as her mother is alive, she will be as supportive as possible.

With both daughters in agreement about letting Melanie choose her own life and death, she seems more at peace. "Tell me how it's going to be," Melanie implores me. "I want to know what I'm up against along the way. Pull no punches, either—tell it like it is. You're going to be my guide on this journey."

This opens the door for me to share how she is being affected by the decrease in appetite and intake, how she is getting weaker, requiring more equipment and more care. Some people want only the next page talked about, but Melanie wants the whole story.

"I'm reading this book about the pioneers on the Oregon Trail and I see my dying as a trip similar to the one they took. They went into a place unknown to them as I am doing. I need you to tell me the signs along this path and help me to interpret them."

I tell her that each person is different, but there are some commonalities and I will be open with her about those. We talk about decline and pain and how we will work together as new symptoms arise.

Returning from a week's vacation, I am told Melanie is declining significantly and asking for her 'guide.' On arriving at her bedside, I see a weak smile on a very pale face. She asks: "Where are the signs? I've been looking, but I can't see any. I'm so glad to see you. Please help me."

Loretta is with her, tears filling her eyes, "She is refusing to eat anything, even the things she used to love. She says it hurts so bad to be touched that nobody can even hold her hand."

My heart is saddened though I'm grateful she waited for me to return. Many times when I say goodbye and leave on vacation, it is the final goodbye. But the down side is that she refuses to take pain medication from my substitute. Now, I have her liquid morphine in my hand and she accepts it. With this small dose she finds some relief. There is often a generalized intense discomfort that precedes death and she is experiencing it.

"There," she exclaims with a smile, "that feels so much better. Now, tell me about your trip—you were on Cycle Oregon right?" With her pain under control, she is willing to let Loretta and me bathe her. We snuggle her up with warm fuzzy pajamas.

"Don't go yet, I have something I want to give you—something to remember me by," she says, stopping me at the front door. She offers a brass belt buckle two inches across with a raised image of a young girl holding a flower stem with flowers along the outside of the circle. "I want you to have this—it reminds me of you."

Loretta gives me pictures of Melanie in front of her Peace Rose holding a rose in the same pose as the image on the belt buckle.

Melanie dies in her sleep several days later. She found the guide within herself to lead her home.

Author's notes: Chapter 10
Where are the Signs

Note 1: Melanie has been receiving intravenous fluids but has chosen to discontinue these. Hospice agencies do not encourage intravenous fluids, chemotherapy, transfusions nor radiation but do emphasize comfort measures and symptom management.

Note 2: Many hospice patients express a desire to give away something that will help the hospice nurse to remember them. Melanie showed this with the gift of the buckle.

Note 3: A hospice nurse is often referred to as a midwife to death. She is there to guide much like the obstetrical midwife does for the pregnant woman.

How Do You Know

Does he know I'm here
Can she hear me
Will she wait for me to come
Why do I need to say it's
Okay to go
What if she thinks
I'm telling her to die
Does he want me at his bedside
What do I do if she dies when
 I'm here
Will she say goodbye before she leaves
How do I know he's not hungry
Why does she always look up
Why does he call for his mother
And ask to go home
When will he take his last breath
How do I know she's not in pain
What do I say when he asks
If he is dying
How do I know you are telling me the truth.

I only know what my teachers have told me
Those with whom I've walked
To Death's door.

AVON CALLING

Rubbing Skin-So-Soft lotion on my hands brings back memories of the day I used it for a massage as a present for Mary's eighty-seventh birthday.

At my first meeting with Mary, her daughter Joan blurts out her demands. "You will not give her any morphine, and you'll never tell her she doesn't have to take her pills. Don't ever say she gets things her way—because if she has her way she won't eat, won't walk and won't try to do anything for herself. I know because I've cared for her through two strokes, and she'd have given up each time if I hadn't pushed her to do more." Joan pauses for a deep breath. "If you agree, you can get started with Mom."

I acknowledge Joan's needs, knowing that her real concern is not wanting to lose her mother. "I will do my best, but sometimes the best laid plans go awry." I turn to Mary and smile, "My job is to make you comfortable, pain-free and to help Joan give you the best quality of life possible. Sometimes people actually get better on hospice, and I have the privilege of discharging them from our service."

Joan quickly explains, "Mom is recovering from pneumonia after her third stroke. The other strokes were not this bad. This time she needed to go back to the hospital when she choked on some food and got a bad case of pneumonia. We're using a thickening powder—Thicket, I think it's called—right now so she won't choke again. She doesn't like it."

"Coffee is not coffee," Mary adds, somewhat defiantly. Then she looks over at me and winks with a smile, "Well, it's…" she pauses, searching for the right word.

"Yes, coffee is the one exception I make since she won't drink it if I add thickener to it. But she always sits up at the table when she drinks her coffee," Joan explains as Mary smiles. "And I watch her closely."

"You know, I was told by the nurse who admitted Mom to hospice that you believe the patient should get what she wants," Joan says. "But you see, Mom and I just bought this home together. I came down from northern Canada to care for her. I want to share this home and spend as much time as possible with her."

Mary smiles and adds her comment with the sentence unfinished, "Yes, this is our...Welcome."

"She has difficulty completing sentences. It's part of the stroke damage," Joan says somewhat apologetically.

Mary's pills are lined up on the table at our next visit, and Joan asks, "Can we get her pills in liquid form? I've been crushing them and putting them in her food, but she spits them out. She says they taste bad and refuses to swallow them." Mary sits at the table behind Joan, making a face. Her daughter points to untouched scrambled eggs.

"She might eat more if the pills weren't added. I think she spits the pill out because it tastes bitter."

I mention the possibility of another bout of pneumonia if she chokes on a pill, a bite of food or even a swallow of coffee.

Joan responds, "I know it is a risk and may happen, but I can't stand to see Mom die without at least trying to force good food on her. She's got two more antibiotic pills to take from her prescription." Seeing my look of surprise she says, "I know people in hospice don't usually take antibiotics, but I want her to finish this course of pills. Your other nurse said it would be all right."

I have learned that families need to do all they can so they can accept the death of their loved one. I say nothing but nod in agreement.

I watch as Mary walks to the sofa with Joan's assistance—she could not have done it alone. She is unable to keep balance due to the stroke and her ongoing weakness.

"Please, come...," Mary invites me to sit next to her as she pats the sofa.

"Would you like some little pillows and a lap blanket?" I ask, seeing how her body leans to the right, "Our volunteers make these," I say taking a small pillow out of my nurse's bag. "These might help to keep you from falling to the right. And this blanket is so warm and fuzzy. I'll be tempted to take this one home if you don't like it."

Mary smiles and puts the soft blanket to her face. She seems more centered with the pillows at her side.

As the visit ends, Joan walks with me to my car and says, "Mom would never want to be seen this way. She's a very proud woman, never wanting others to do what she could do herself. I suppose I should let her go, but I want more time with her. But I think she wants to go be with her family up there." She points upward. I notice tears in her eyes and move to hug her.

"I do feel overwhelmed at times," she says as I release the hug. "My sisters aren't able to come for a couple of weeks. Maybe a hospice aide would help. Not to give her a bath but to stay here for a couple of hours while I get out. I'll mention the idea to Mom. Please check back next visit."

As I drive away, I think of how Mary must be processing all of this—a nurse who says she shouldn't have to eat if she doesn't want to and a daughter who says she must; a nurse who says she shouldn't be made to take pills if she can't swallow and a daughter who says she must. It would be no surprise if Mary feels confused.

When I next see Mary, she is holding a picture of deceased family members in her right hand and another of her daughters as youngsters in the weakened left hand. I see a smile as she moves her eyes back and forth as if being between her parents and her children.

Daughter Joan is in the kitchen quietly crying, trying not to be seen by Mary. "If only I hadn't gotten mad at her," she sobs as I give her a hug. "If only I hadn't lost my patience, maybe she wouldn't want to leave us. I spoke sharply to her as we were getting her dressed this morning. I feel so bad. Why did I yell at her?"

"You're working hard, caring for a loved one, Joan," I say reassuringly. "Your mom's not holding that against you. As I see it, she is being torn between those who held her and those she held. She knows she'll be joining her parents, but I'm sure she's sad to leave you three girls. Remember, this is a process, and it will take time to accept and adjust."

I look at Mary who is pointing to her father. She starts to cry. Then moving her eyes and a finger to the picture of three young girls, she tries to say their names: "Jenny," "Joan" and "Kathy." The names come out of her mouth deliberately and slowly. Tears continue to flow down her cheeks.

I bring Joan to her and hold their hands. "You must have some very good memories of your family, Mary. Your girls are fortunate to have such a loving mother. I'm so honored to be here with the two of you,"

Joan wipes her tears and begins telling a story of their youth when her mother visited California and decided she would bring her kids there to live.

"Dad didn't want to leave New York, but my mom, she was the boss, and so California is where we ended up," she says laughingly as she looks at her mother.

I listen, intrigued and laughing, with both Mary and her daughter as they tell stories of the past. I see a distant look in Mary's eyes and check to see if Joan is noticing it.

Instead Joan quickly turns the conversation to a party. "We are going to have a great big bash for Mom's 87th birthday. I hope you can come. My sisters and their children will all be here. It'll be a week from Friday. Jenny is coming from San Francisco and Kathy from Alaska. There'll be about 40 people here. It's going to be fun, isn't it, Mom?"

A look of concern crosses Mary's face, "Please cgrrhhr. I don't wwwwwsss."

Joan interprets, "She doesn't want a big party. I'm sure she's a bit nervous with all those people coming here to this small house…but everyone wants the chance to see you, Mom and this way it'll all be at one time." Turning to me, she asks, "Will you come?"

"I'd love to come and meet your family. You're going to be real busy, planning and cooking for all those people." I pause looking to see if there is any resentment. "What are you making?

Joan replies, "Lasagna, using Mom's recipe."

Over the next few visits we order new equipment to make caring for Mary easier. When Mary falls trying to get out of bed to go to the bathroom, I suggest a bedside commode and an alarm that will sound when she tries to get out of bed alone. I also order a reclining wheelchair, thinking it might be helpful, allowing for fewer transfers from bed to chair and back. Mary can sit upright or let it tilt back for sleeping during the day.

A bath aide has been helping and providing some respite for a week now. Now Joan can feel more at ease taking her time to shop. She won't have to worry about leaving her mother alone.

At my next visit Mary seems almost in another world talking about a dream. I have brought Native American flute music since she no longer enjoys the television programs she's loved in the past. Her eyes beam when I play the Carlos Nakai CD.

"It sounds like it's from…" Mary slowed down and couldn't finish her sentence, but points up and smiles generously at me. "I like it!" she clearly says to me. "Leave it, please."

Joan tells me her sisters are due tomorrow to prepare for the party, but she has concerns. "Mom is talking like she's not here. She's talking in the third person saying 'SHE' doesn't want a big party and that 'SHE' doesn't want to go outside. I wonder if that music is causing her to want to leave us before her party."

I shake my head. But when I listen to Mary, I hear the same thing, as if she has disembodied herself and is referring to someone else.

"She's come a long way…" she says as she points at the picture of herself as a toddler.

"Mary," I ask, "is there anything you'd like for your birthday? Can I bring you something? Or how about a massage? We have a volunteer massage therapist. Would you like a massage?"

"I've never had a…"she replies, turning to look at me but unable to say with the word, massage.

The therapist is booked for several weeks, so the next visit I come prepared to give Mary her massage. I've brought several lotions, candles and some relaxation music.

Mary exclaims, "Oh yeah," when she sees the bottle of Skin-So-Soft lotion.

Joan explains, "Mom used to sell Avon products, and she loves that smell."

Mary falls asleep after the massage. Joan and I step out of her room, hearing seascape music playing softly. Joan suddenly turns and hugs me.

"Thank you so very much for your gift and your love. Mom really loves you. Things are getting hard even with my sisters here. We're trying to get everything ready for the party. You're coming, aren't you?" Joan asks quietly.

I nod knowing that Joan has finally agreed to give Mary only what she wants to eat and she still gets her coffee without the thickener in it. We have gradually discontinued the medications because, even in the liquid form, she spits them out.

Before leaving I return to Mary's room to get her blood pressure. Mary opens her eyes, smiles and falls right back asleep. When I report the perfect reading to Joan she hugs me again, reassured that no harm is being done withholding the blood pressure medication.

The birthday visit for me is to be only a meet-and-greet of her family, but I know many people will have questions, some no one can answer. I get there just before the cake is served. Mary is asking to go to bed. Joan and her sisters gather the family around the bed to sing Happy Birthday. Later they return to say goodbyes as they leave for the day. After the last person tells her goodbye, Mary immediately falls asleep. She never gets out of that bed again.

That final birthday weekend is filled with family plans since the daughters are still in town. Everybody wants to spend time with Mary, but she isn't up to entertaining or being entertained. She is busy doing her own thing, and everyone understands.

Joan calls on Monday telling me I'm needed. "Mom's not doing well. We haven't done what the night nurse told us to because my sisters are afraid if we do it, we'll kill her. Why do we have to give her more medicine?" Joan asks. "Shouldn't that anxiety medicine settle her down? We gave her one dose, but then she woke up and became very agitated. I'm afraid she's going to crawl out of this bed," Joan sounds very frustrated. "She keeps saying she has to leave. We don't understand. Can you come right out?"

"Yes," I assure her. "But give her a dose now, and we'll talk when I get there. Your sisters will be okay with that, right?"

I explain the need for medication as I walk down the hall followed by Joan and her sisters. "It is necessary to give her the prescribed amount every six hours because if the effects wear off, she'll get antsy again. Even if she can't swallow, this medicine can be placed under her tongue with the dropper." Demonstrating, I administer another dose of the Ativan and say, " See how easy it is? And another thing, remember how Mary loved having a massage the other day? Let's rub the Skin-So-Soft Lotion on her arms and legs."

I position the three daughters at Mary's arm and legs. I hold her other arm and begin to rub in the lotion. "This way each of you will be touching her, soothing her with her favorite smell. I have a feeling she'll love it. Do you realize how important this is to her? The ones she gave life to are with her in her death and her passage into heaven." I then invite each to share a loving memory of their mother. As they share, Mary's breathing begins to slow, and she appears very calm.

Joan smiles as she continues to caress her mother. "Now, instead of Avon calling, it's God calling."

After the rubbing and soothing, Mary begins breathing with long breaths, almost like a moan or an *ah...a...a...ah* sound.

I explain about the *aah* sound, "It's very hard to hold your breath while saying *aah*. Try it." I tell each of them to take a big breath. "Now, let it go with an *ahh* sound. This is the sound of your mother letting go."

Everyone takes another deep breath and sighs with a common *ahh..h..h.* sound. Everyone in the room knows Mary's spirit is leaving. She takes one last long breath and is gone.

Author's notes: Chapter 11
Avon Calling

Note 1: When I admitted Mary to hospice, I offered assistance and additional help. Joan didn't want it at that time but accepted a volunteer so she could have some free time. Eventually Mary needed more help with her bathing. Volunteers are trained and placed by a coordinator in accord with the family and patient's needs.

Note 2: There is twenty-four hour coverage for continuity of care. Case manager nurses will leave a report for the night nurse that covers complex or actively dying patients.

Note 3: I demonstrated to Joan and her sisters that holding their breath stops the breath flow, but letting it go with an "*aaah*" sound opens the breathing and represents a letting go. Joan and her sisters were in the vigil phase during the weekend. This very hard time often requires the support of a chaplain or a nurse.

Note 4: "Heartwork" is a phrase used to denote the private time for soul or spirit work needed before letting go can occur.

I wrote the following letters to a friend who is dying and his wife. They demonstrate the concept of "Heartwork" and "Vigil."

Dear one:

Your note was very heartfelt, especially the comment you made, "A lot going on which reduces me to tears."

This is so very true in all aspects of your vigil. And sweet friend, this is what this is--regardless of how you frame it. You and I both know this is the time of him letting go and you letting him go.

His physical "home" is no longer able to contain his spirit. His body is likened to the house in disrepair and unable to accommodate the resident any longer. It is time to move on to a bigger and better "place." But right now he is where I describe as the place between here and there. It's like a line is drawn on the ground and he is moving back and forth from side to side. At times he might be present for you and others and at other times he has already left to another plane. Our job now is to hold him in love as his inner spirit allows his full release there.

The task for him is to now do the final "heartwork" necessary for that release.

It hurts us as loved ones and witnesses to see our precious one in the place he is in but knowing that we must trust the process with no holding, no expectations and no regrets. This then is the vigil—and it takes as long as it takes.

I have been asked so many times "How long will this take?" when the loved one is where your husband is. My response is always the same: "No one has that answer—no doctor, nurse, friend, caregiver or hospice nurse. When I became a hospice nurse, I wasn't issued a fortuneteller's glass ball to predict this time accurately. If I said a month or two weeks, it would certainly be a day or two or even three months."

However the difficulty with pain control and the fact that he's telling you that he hurts all over his body gives me clues that death is not a long ways off. Usually the process is that people start showing a lack of interest in food or activity, eating less, not wanting to drink water. There is no pain associated with not eating, though many are concerned about the hunger. Now the emphasis is on nurturing with love and providing comfort, safety and pain relief. When you related of his earlier desire to get exercise I got the clue that his pain wasn't limiting his activity. But now I hear you say he is more confused and unable to move without some degree of pain.

The term *anam cara* is given to the person who in Celtic tradition is a soul friend. John O'Donohue, poet, priest and teacher, wrote a book titled *Anam Cara*. In this book he clarifies this to include the one person who accompanies the dying to his transition or the midwife. Since your lives have flowed together for 30 years and you recognize his process as inevitable, you are the *anam cara* for him. You are holding this vigil for him. You will walk him to that point of death beyond which you may not enter.

I also know that he may choose, on some level to protect you from his final breath by taking leave of his body when you are not there. Please know that his happens even to the most committed folks. Promises are made and then at the end, a choice may be made differently with the letting go happening when the loved one has left the room. Stories are told of death occurring at the moment a bathroom break is taken.

The tears you are shedding are the sweetest part of death, though the hardest to endure. I trust you have established a dear friend or hospice worker that is there for you personally and not in the words of email but someone who holds you and allows these tears to flow. You are doing the anticipatory grieving now. There will, of course, be much later, but please be at peace with those tears at this time.

Remember, there is little you can do now except be present as he completes this phase of his journey. The desire to "do" something is natural but now little can be done except make him comfortable.

Also remember there are many people who are holding both you and him in their energy fields so that each of our higher purposes will be met.

I love you and hold you tight to my heart. I light a candle each morning as I meditate.

A letter to my friend who is letting go:

Dear one;

I know how you are hurting right now. I know you are longing in many ways for release from this pain and suffering. Dear one, it will come in its time. Right now you are right where you are supposed to be. The work that's going on inside you is called heartwork by those of us who are well-versed in the dying process. I know that you, as a dying man, are very sensitive to those you love. You want them to be at peace before you leave this plane. So you are taking the time necessary to achieve the goal of letting go in the perfect time. Your sweet wife is not yet ready to see you go or you would have already left. You are telling her in so many ways that you are spending a large portion of your time in that other plane, that you are seeing things nobody but you can see and are preparing to leave her.

You were quite clear to me when you related in your dream you are driving a car that's built by the Source for only you. And Dear one that is true: what's happening to you is only for your eyes. You can't possibly share it with your world thoroughly, though your love is writing these fine accounts of what's going on. You and I both realize that they are for her purposes to help her get in time with the music that's playing in your heart.

I know there is a lovely melody playing in the background of this process and at times you are already in your heaven. For right now you are surrounded by love, held in the hearts of those who sang and danced with you in your life. You are loved and indeed are LOVE—the fullest expression of it possible while being in your body. I also know there is pain right now—I venture a guess that it is miserable at times. I am sorry for that and know that there is a solution to this and it might mean release from this physical body your spirit is residing in right now. For, you see, my dear friend, this body is but a house, moving into need for major repair—so major that it is wiser to move to a better home than to stay here and try to make those repairs. Your spirit wants to soar fly high above this earthly plane.

Peace to you on your journey,

Lovingly,
Your friend

PART THREE

Forgiveness

As I sit on the top of Dog Mountain, I look at beauty all around me. I see Mt. Hood on my left, Mt. Adams and Mt. St. Helens on my right and a hillside of Nature's most magnificent bouquet of yellow balsam root and purple lupines. A pair of swallowtail butterflies circles above my head in an ascending pattern against a backdrop of a blue sky dotted with fluffy white clouds. My gaze lands on the river stretching below me like a silver thread winding its way to the sea. I am reminded of a poem by Thich Nhat Hanh I once read to a man named Floyd as he was dying from lung cancer. A smile spreads across my face as I remember Floyd's story.

Floyd is of Japanese descent, and he lives alone at eighty-one. He has remained independent and active until recently.

"Yeah, the saddest parts of my life were when my wife died two years ago—gosh, I miss her—and when my brother died fighting in the war. My furniture business downtown was seized, and we were sent to Idaho for the internment camp. My younger brother signed up for the army and was killed before our family was released from that camp." Floyd tells this story early in my time with him. "But that was then; now I have my two dogs and a large beautiful family. I used to go fishing and mushroom picking—we sure loved those big mushrooms I'd bring home. I don't have any energy to do that now."

Hearing stories are an important part of bonding and getting to know the person I will be sitting beside as he ends his life story. Floyd loves to talk, pausing to puff his cigarette and form smoke rings.

"My big worry," he says after several visits, "is that I will become unable to care for myself. I've done it all after my wife died, and I hate becoming dependent. I have four kids, and they are all very busy with life and work. I don't want them to take care of me. I've heard about that pill and wonder if it is possible for you to bring it out to me? Not now of course, but when I need it before I get to be a burden. Could you see about getting it for me?" He pauses with a faraway look in his eyes, "I'd really like to see my wife."

"The Oregon Death with Dignity Act that passed is not as easy to access as you might think," I reply. I've had several hospice patients asking on my first visit if I've brought 'the pill' for them to take. "The bill you're talking about isn't a pill but is a process of several evaluations with wait periods. It requires a lot of jumping through hoops and time, allowing many days to pass before another exam. I can get you information on it and give you a contact number. You'll need to think it over and discuss that with your family. I'm sure they're going to have input on the subject." He nods understanding. "Let's talk some more about this later, okay?"

Over the next few weeks, Floyd begins to adjust to his decreasing strength and weakness, allowing me to order a hospital bed. "But I'm not going to use it until I have to," he vows, "I need room for Tippy and Sammy to sleep with me."

At the next visit he is using it along with the two Pomeranians. I smile, remembering how resistant he was.

He speaks forcefully trying to be in control, "If I have to die, you'd think I could do it on my terms, wouldn't you? I mean why does it have to take so long?"

"I don't know why—but I think it has to do with the flow. We can't rush the river of life. You're right, sometimes life and death suck. When I first started visiting, you struggled with the lung cancer diagnosis and the doctor's prognosis of less than six months, and now you're having difficulty with the time it takes. I understand. I'd like to meet your daughter soon so I can give her support during this process. Does she come over often to see you?"

"Yes, Janice was just here asking about you. I'll ask her to come for next time."

At the next visit, Floyd opens the conversation with his daughter next to him, "I don't want you to miss work for me, Janice. I'm becoming a bother and I don't like it."

"Dad, this is what we all want to do," Janice responds gently. "We know hospice can help a little, but the boys and I have made a plan. We're sharing so nobody carries the entire load—and you're not a bother! We love you."

I respond, "Do you remember the Green Stamps—S&H, I think they were. Janice, maybe you're too young to know about them. Remember, Floyd, shopping where they were given with the sales slip? We'd take them home and paste them in the books, redeeming them when the book was full. Getting exciting things we couldn't afford was great. I remember how we as a family were able to go to Disneyland when it first opened because of them.

Both of them nod their heads. Floyd says, looking at Janice, "We'll never forget that ugly lamp Mom got with them, will we? I thought it was useless…But what's this got to do with us now?"

"Well," I answer, "if you were given a stamp for each time you helped one of your children—like holding up the bike for Janice to learn to ride or teaching each of your four children to drive or staying up late when they were out after curfew—and after you got that stamp you put it in a book, just how many books would you have filled by now?" I look over at Janice who is smiling. "Consider all those books you would have filled, including ones for your grandkids and nieces and nephews— as being used now to justify these kids giving their time and energy to make sure you're well-cared for."

Janice is crying and smiling at the same time. "Dad, she's right. Caring for you is our gift to you. We were robbed of that opportunity with Mom because she died suddenly. But we want to do this, trust me," she says, bowing her head a little as if to thank me.

"I have a green stamp book," Floyd adds as if he can defer the attention by redirecting the conversation. "Please get it, Janice, it's in the old dresser in the spare room."

"Why, do you want it? Are you going to sell it to her?" Janice questions but gets up to find it.

"Hell, yes, I'm selling it to her. It must be worth $2.00," he laughingly replies and then winks at me. "I guess I understand about the kids helping me, but it's hard to accept."

He hands me the book when Janice returns, "Now you can have this to show people who can't remember using the stamps! It's free to you today. Thanks for the story."

Floyd declines very slowly and once again questions why it's taking so long for him to die. "I've got everything in order; I've given away all my money. I've even found a grandson who will take Tippy and Sammy and give them a good home. Why? Why? Why can't I just die and get it over with? I miss my wife so very much."

"Listen, Floyd, I don't have the answers. It's a mystery, like much of life. I brought a poem I'd like to read to you—it's about the flow of a river. Would that be okay?" I ask knowing nothing is going to answer his age-old question.

"*The Story of a River*, from a collection of poems by Thich Nhat Hanh, is about a small stream excited to be one with the ocean. She wishes to forgo any obstacles or delays along the way but instead, faces lessons that cause her to appreciate the time it takes." As I start to read, I note he is making himself comfortable and settling in to listen.

After reading several pages, he stops me. "Is this supposed to be about me?" Floyd questions, but leans forward into the story.

I finish with a statement when the river realizes that she doesn't have to rush to become what she already was—water.

Floyd speaks quietly, "Thank you for reading that. I think you're saying I ask too many questions about when I will die, right? Do others ask why they're not dying fast enough? I do wonder why I'm still here. Is this story supposed to help me get into the flow? 'Cuz if it is, I'm not liking it. But I'll try and be more patient. I guess I'll have to learn to live until I die and not expect it in my timing."

He blows a puff of smoke my way and grins, "Just checking your reaction, especially since you don't smoke." We have had an ongoing discussion about smoking and especially his blowing of smoke-rings. He acts proud of himself.

Unfortunately Floyd has bumped his foot on the wheelchair and a sore has developed that isn't healing. It has become quite painful, so when I start giving him liquid pain medication for this pain, he asks, "Is this a part of the flow?"

I nod and continue the bandaging I've been doing since the wound started draining.

He's becoming more dependent on his children, requiring twenty-four hour care. The four children alternate staying nights with him. He no longer asks the timing question. His family follows my suggestion to make him king and give him all he wants to eat. I find his friends there talking, laughing, playing cards with him as much as he is able. He orders a box of persimmons through the mail to give to friends and family. He insists I try one when he gives it to me. I comment on its sweetness, unlike other persimmons I've tasted.

"I've been honored to meet your beautiful family," I say to Floyd one visit. His two boys are lifting him into the wheelchair that he had so vehemently refused for so long.

"Aren't my kids wonderful to me?" Floyd asks after they get him settled. He asks for a cigarette. No one criticizes him for smoking, but they watch him more closely since he fell asleep smoking last week.

Floyd quickly declines, requiring increasing levels of pain control. Hospice aides come to provide respite for his family.

Surrounded by children and grandchildren, enveloped in love, Floyd dies in his sleep several nights later, joining that flow of life back to its source.

Author's notes: Chapter 12
The Green Stamps

Note 1: The frequency of the R.N. visits is determined by patient need. When Floyd's wound required daily visits to change his dressing, I went daily. I was able to decrease my schedule of visits to weekly or twice weekly.

Note 2: In 1997, Oregon was the first state to vote in the *Death with Dignity* Act. There are time-consuming guidelines to follow to qualify for the medications. The term *Doctor Assisted Suicide* has been changed to *Physician Aid in Dying* by most professionals.

Note 3: Floyd was interested in hastening his death because he perceived he was a burden to his family.

"I don't want to go anywhere else other than right here—ever! I'll kill myself if you put me in a nursing home," Tom says in his strong Jersey accent. I've been in his son's home for less than ten minutes, but he's made his point clear about relocating. His son Sam and daughter-in-law Jody have brought him home from the Veteran's hospital after one final treatment for pancreatic cancer. They've moved their son downstairs to allow Tom to spend his dying time with them.

"I'm finally home with my family, and here's where I want to die. But I'm not dying yet. I want to have a garden—I want to see it plowed, planted, watch the seedlings come up, water and harvest them. I've made a plan, and Sam is going to help make it work," Tom says. Though he's very thin and weak, he appears enthusiastic as he points to the backyard. "I gotta make a big garden with lots of vegetables to give back to my family. I know they've given up a lot." He smiles and continues, "Look here, they've even put a fridge in here for my beer. And this dog, Blacky, is my grandson's dog, but he wants to stay here with me."

"Man, you're pretty lucky to have your own fridge where all you have to do is turn over for that Bud," I say laughing with him.

"I'm willing to do what I can to help keep you here," I tell him and Jody. "We have a lot of support for him and for you as family. An aide can help with bathing or bed linen change. A social worker will be calling to make a visit. She'll be a great person to talk to all of you, including your son. "

"Tom's got that big sore on his butt—Would you teach me to change the bandage?" Jody's reminding me of the bedsore, so I look at it and change the dressing. I tell her that I'll bring supplies and teach her how to do it on the next visit.

Jody takes me aside as we leave Tom's room, "Dad's had nothing but problems all his life. He's been pretty brutal to his kids. He had a horrible childhood. He had several marriages, drank a lot and now can't care for himself. My husband's sister tried to take care of him, but he was so demanding that she burned out quickly. My husband, Sam, said he would only take this on with my support and help from hospice. We have friends who swear by hospice. One person said they got a lot of support from you as his father was dying."

She pauses to think before continuing, "About my husband Sam, I don't think he's going to talk to anybody but me. He hides his emotions. But I'll be sure to tell him whatever you and I talk about."

I've seen how gentle Jody is with Tom. She speaks positively of her ability to manage him. "I told him we will keep a fridge in here for his beer, but we'll need to limit them when he needs more pain medication. He's not too happy about that thought. He's always done a lot of drinking. I think that's been the problem with Cindy, the daughter he was staying with."

I tell her I understand and sense her relief in our goodbye hug.

When I come for my next visit Tom tells me, "My son's going to make a door over there so I can go out and watch my garden grow." He points to the back wall. "And then we, or I should say they, will begin to clear the back yard."

He pauses, so I gesture for him to turn over, "I get what you want—you want me over so you can change that dressing on my butt." This is in response to my fourth request that he let me take care of the sore he got while in the hospital. These often occur with weight loss and limited movement in bed. Poor circulation around bony parts doesn't help either.

His wound requires the dressing to be changed every three days, so my visits are that frequent. "I'll stop coming this often after I can teach Jody to do the change. You'd really help yourself out by turning from side-to-side at least every two hours," I advise him. "It won't get well and will probably get worse if you don't change position."

"Oh yeah," he replies, "but you can't know what a bother it is. It interrupts my TV program, makes smoking hard and I can't get to my beer when I'm on my other side. And I can't eat there, either." He reaches for a Budweiser from his fridge. "But I'll try harder but guess that's all I can do—is to try. Jody is doing a great job."

Jody comes in to watch as I change the large bandage. "He doesn't want to turn, but I tell him we won't be able to get him outside to the garden if this sore doesn't heal," she says to me and then directly at Tom. "I told you, I'd tell Sharon. You better behave," she says in a stern voice. Then she laughs with Tom and me. "I'm sure I can handle the dressing changes.

Tom takes his own pills until one day his family can't wake him and Jody calls me. When I get there to check, I see the evening's pain pill is gone from the pillbox. Tom is sleeping soundly from the double dose. No harm done this time. Now Jody takes charge of the pill box and doles them out on schedule, leaving the night dose on the bedside table to be taken after the David Letterman show.

The rainy season drags on, but Tom continues to be excited about the garden. He's drawing sketches of what he wants planted where.

Several visits later, he points at the newly-installed door leading to 'his' garden space and says, "Sam just finished yesterday. It's going to be so good. He's building the deck next. Once the sun comes out, it'll be great sitting out there. But what's with this weather?" he says, scowling. "Is summer ever going to happen here?"

"Would you tell him he must stop smoking in bed?" Jody asks when she comes in.

She turns to Tom, "Last night, you fell asleep with a lit cigarette and burned my sheets. We can't have that—your grandson is sleeping right below."

I recently switched the pain pill to a patch because Tom wasn't getting good control with the pills. Now he's getting relief but falls asleep easily, sometimes with a drink and a cigarette in his hands. "We're in a tough place, Tom. We want you to feel good but to also be responsible—falling asleep with a lit cigarette is dangerous. What can we do to help you enjoy life and still be safe, especially with the smoking?" I ask. I really want him to give a solution instead of forcing mine on him.

"My son's already said that Jody's going to be in charge of the cigs and I'll only smoke when someone is in the room with me. That's cool with me," he answers somewhat begrudgingly. Then he turns to Jody. "Can I have a smoke while she's here? She'll watch to make sure I don't fall asleep." He looks at me and winks, "Let's take care of that business down there first. Jody's been doing it and says it's almost well. Yeah for Jody. She says that sore is improving—maybe next time you can take a look at it."

"I've been thinking," he says as soon as Jody brings him his smoke and leaves, "I've done a lot of bad things in my life. I've been a bad guy, in and out of jail and I've caused lots of pain to my wives, to my kids and even my friends. Being here in this bed, waiting for the sun to come out so I can plant my garden, has given me lots of time to think about my life. You know what I mean?" He looks right into my eyes as he speaks.

"Yes, I do," I respond. You want to talk about that?

Drawing a big puff off the unfiltered Camel, he says, "Yeah, I think I owe a lot of people apologies. I wish I could go back and talk to those I've hurt, but now I can't. I'd like to make it up to my daughter and some of my friends. I always went around with a chip on my shoulder daring anybody to knock it off. I've been responsible for several people getting hurt—I mean I didn't do it, but I was the reason behind it," he speaks with all bravado gone. "Is there any way you can help me?"

"I can ask the social worker to come and a chaplain is available also. Would you like them to visit with you about this? Should I call your daughter Cindy and see how she's doing?" I ask quietly.

" I don't want a chaplain. He'll just try to save my soul. I'm okay with a social worker; didn't I meet her before? And let's call Cindy later. I'll tell you when. I think she's going come out for a visit. Not sure when that'll be."

"You know, Tom, maybe you could write a letter to those you've harmed," I suggest.

"No, I don't write well. I can't sit up for very long. The pain in my belly gets worse when I do that," he explains.

"There's another thing used for forgiveness work—and that's what you're talking about," I say. "I have a hand-held tape recorder. It's voice-activated so it shuts itself off when nothing is being said, like if you fall asleep as you're talking. Would you like me to bring that and send apologies in tape form?" I ask him.

"That'd be good. Yes, I think I could do that. I can think of several people I'd ask forgiveness from. I want to make one for my family here, telling them how much I thank them and then for my friends back east," he replies with a smile. "I'm sorry I'm such a pain for Jody. But let me make this perfectly clear," he says speaking as though he's now changing direction, "understand, I'm not dying. I'm really getting stronger, so I can go outside with that garden."

I smile, knowing very well the value of a goal, especially when on hospice.

The weather begins to clear, the deck is finished and I greet Tom on a sunny day. He's outside sitting in a chair, looking over a freshly rototilled yard. "This is perfect," he says pointing, "my beans will be over there, my tomatoes here and my squash over there so they can climb the fence. Isn't this great? I got it all planned. I'm so proud of myself."

I smile, happy to see him enjoying himself.

"By the way, can you bring me some more tapes? I finished that one. It feels good to be able to talk instead of write," he says grinning.

Several weeks later he asks, "Would you like to see my garden?" I note that the beans are filling out the strings and the squash are blossoming. I hold on to his arm, helping him to the walker. As he goes between the rows, he comments, "See how beautiful it is? You know there's one thing I ask myself; Why didn't I get more life insurance so my family could have got something from this cancer? I regret that. I'd then have so much more to give," he states matter-of-factly. Then, as if he puts the train in reverse, he asks, "Would you like some zucchini? We have so many of them that we don't know what to do with them. Maybe you can take some to the office?" He sits on the edge of the raised bed with a big grin on his face and starts pulling out radishes, "I don't think I've ever been happier."

Tom goes outside as much as possible as summer slides into early autumn, but now he's pretty limited, needing to be lifted into a wheelchair. "I've got these six tapes done. This one is for my family—I feel good about doing it. You see, I couldn't do just one tape like you suggested—I have too many people to apologize to." He holds up the tapes. "Did Jody tell you my daughter Cindy's coming next week? It'll be so good to see her. I want you to meet her."

Jody's calling from the kitchen as I leave, so I stop to chat. On the counter are several big pans of bright red, ripe tomatoes that she's stuffing into canning jars.

"I am so glad you've been able to come regularly to see him. He really likes you. It's been great having his pain under control," she says. "We'll be gone this weekend. Cindy will be staying here with Dad."

When I visit after that weekend, Cindy has already left for New Jersey, so I am unable to visit with her, but Tom's beaming with happiness. "I had a good time with her. She liked the veggies from my garden and was very proud of what we've done. I had a good talk with her and sent some tapes home with her. I want my son to play the one I've made for them after I go. You can take your recorder back. I'm through with it. Thanks for the loan."

Several days later Jody calls about Tom: "He's acting real strange. He's talking out of his head. Can you come out to see him, please—and could you come quickly?" She asks.

"Hi Tom," I say as I walk in the room.

"Dad, Sharon's here."

"I'm burning up in my bed," Tom starts talking fast. "My parents are here. They're talking to me. I can't talk to them or I'll be joining them. I've got to stay here. I can't go." There is a agitated look in his eyes. I look across the bed at Jody and sense she understands that Tom is near death.

When we step out of Tom's room I ask Jody, "Is Sam aware of how close his dad is to death? I know you know, because we've spent a lot of time talking about this, but I haven't spent much time with your husband. Is he home today?"

"No, but I think he's knows. He's watched the decline over the past few days. I'll call him. His office is nearby."

I return to Tom. His temperature is 101 and his pulse is fast, but he has calmed down. I put on a CD of peaceful harp music and start talking softly.

"It's okay, Tom. You've done a good job. You've made a great garden and given lots of love to these folks here. If your mom and dad are calling you, it's fine to go with them," Now I'm taking his blood pressure and listening to his heart.

Jody interrupts us. "Can you talk to Sam? He drove like a race car driver to get here."

"Sure, stay here with Tom for a few minutes," I say and then to him. "Tom, I'm going to be with your son and then we'll be in to see you. Okay?"

I go down the hallway to the kitchen, where I explain to Sam what I've seen and what I think is going on.

"You think it's not far off, don't you? I checked him before I left for work, and I thought then he wouldn't make it through the day. You think so too, don't you? Should we get my son home from school? We told him we'd make sure he had a chance to say goodbye," Sam speaks in a rush, running his thoughts all together.

"I think the most important thing right now is for you to be with him. Let him know you are here. I can't tell how long he has, but he is close. About Tommy, I can't give you that answer. I could probably get a social worker out here to talk with him if you think she might help," I'm trying to reassure him. He accepts a proffered hug and begins to tear up and pushes me away. "Now is probably a good time to tell him you love him and give him permission to go with his parents. He just told me that he saw them but couldn't go with them."

Sam objects. "But wouldn't that be like telling him to die?"

"No," I reply, "you're telling him of your love for him and that you'll all be okay. It's like saying, 'we know you have to go and we'll miss you, but we'll remember you.'"

I check to ensure he has enough medication to last the night before I leave. I'm sure they will need both pain med liquid and the anti-anxiety medication.

"Now, Jody, you remember what to do if Tom dies before morning," I ask.

"Yes, I'm supposed to call hospice, and they'll take care of everything, right? You guys don't have to make a visit; isn't that what you said?"

"That's right. But remember— tell the nurse when you call in if you'd like a visit. We are more than willing to come out, but don't want to push ourselves in during this very private time. But I want to thank you for letting me get to know Tom and your family. I consider that a privilege," I give these final instructions quietly and leave after a hug.

Tom's name is listed in the morning report of deaths that occurred during the night. No nursing visit was made. When I called Jody, she said her son had stayed home from school, and she'd arranged for a counselor to spend time with him.

The family was well prepared, and I'm sure they truly enjoyed the harvest from Tom's garden.

Author's notes: Chapter 13
Garden of Hope and Forgiveness

Note 1: Tom's wounds were due to poor nutrition, weight loss and a lack of turning. Many people on hospice get buttock or coccyx wounds due to this, and the wounds can be very difficult to heal. I taught Jody, his daughter-in-law, to change the bandage because it had a tendency to fall off.

Note 2: By providing Tom with a method to seek forgiveness, we helped him feel complete. Gardening allowed him a means to give back to his family.

Note 3: The hospice social worker, trained in grief counseling, was able to offer support to Tom's grandsons.

PART FOUR

Acceptance and Letting Go

"Wanna see all my angels? I've got them all over. I've been collecting them for years," Helen announces right after I introduce myself. "I'm the keeper of the angels—that's what my grandkids call me." There are angels as pictures, as statues, as mobiles, even an angel doll with filament threads that turn colors from red to green to blue. "My whole family knows what presents to get me for Christmas, birthdays or Mother's Day. I love my angels!"

"I may be 72 years old with cancer, but I'm not dying yet and I'm not giving up my Bingo. So don't plan on visiting me on Thursdays 'cuz I won't be here. And I plan to keep going as long as I can. It's only two blocks from here and Colleen, my daughter, likes to go too. Sometimes I even win money, maybe $5.00."

I like patients with spunk and those who are determined to live as fully as possible. And she has both. From that moment on, she becomes a favorite of mine. I look forward to each Wednesday visit with her.

Helen, in the final stages of lung cancer, lives in a rented house with her daughter Colleen who's left her job in order to care for her. Obviously, she's enjoying taking her mother to bingo.

"I am so worried about my daughters," Helen responds when I ask how she's doing. This spunky lady is more concerned about her family than she is about her own condition. "I don't know what's going to happen with my daughter Pat. She's supposed to have stomach surgery. And that granddaughter, Ellie, I just can't understand why she does what she does. Kids these days, my oh my. My kids would have never done what she's doing—using drugs and all. And there's my son, Dan, who lives in Bend. He divorcing for the third time—what's a mother to do?" I can't answer this question. I can only listen.

Helen enjoys telling me the origin of each angel I see. Colleen has made a showcase of shelves stacked to display all of her prize figurines.

"How are we going to keep Mom from going to the bingo hall?" Colleen asks one day. "She's more tired. Last night she woke up coughing and couldn't get back to sleep. Then she kept me awake for hours, talking about my daughter, telling me how worried she is about her. Then she started in about my sister Pat. She's afraid Pat will die before she gets surgery. Mom's doesn't want Pat to die before she does."

I know how tired and worried Colleen is as I've never heard her express herself quite like this before. But maybe the lack of sleep is to blame. This daughter is generally very patient and kind as she talks about her mother. The stress of caregiving is tremendous. I mention that a volunteer might allow her to take care of herself by getting away at least once a week. I explain that oxygen and a hospital bed could help as well.

With approval from Helen and Colleen, I ask for portable tanks. I also order a wheelchair and a bed with hand controls so Helen can raise her head when she has trouble breathing.

After the equipment is situated, Helen tells me of her progress. "It sure was nice to breathe as I was yelling 'bingo' yesterday. I couldn't have done that last week. Thanks for that small wheelchair; it made it easier to get in and out of the house. And I won $5.00, so I was happy."

Helen's difficulty breathing has eased somewhat, but she still worries about her family. There are some things equipment can't help—and this is one of them, I think as I sit at my desk. I look up, seeing a beautiful small resin stone with an angel in it lying on a shelf. This is perfect for her. It'll be her worry angel.

"Helen, I have something for you. Have you ever heard of worry stones?" I ask on my next visit. "They were popular years ago. They had a thumb indentation to rub when worries haunt the stone holder. Well, I found the perfect one for you. It's not exactly a stone but can serve the same purpose."

As I hand the angel stone to her, I tell her that the angel will listen to all her worries.

"Oh, this is beautiful," Helen exclaims. "I love her. I'm naming her Carol."

"Why?" Colleen asks, coming into the room. "Oh yeah, Carol was a good friend of yours, wasn't she?"

"Yes," Helen starts a story. "Carol was so close to me; we shared everything. We'd sit for hours talking about our kids. She was devastated when her son died at an early age. She was my best friend." Helen sighs, "but she died a couple of months ago. I miss her so much. Yes, this angel will be Carol for me. I'll talk to her about my kids and grandkids. Maybe she'll even give me some answers."

Helen's health begins to deteriorate quickly, so the hospital bed is moved from a bedroom to the living room. She gives up going to Bingo. It's hard enough now for Colleen to get her out of bed to the commode, let alone to the car and back again.

Helen holds the angel stone and says, "I know I can't do anything, but Carol listens. It's so nice to know, whenever I rub this, Carol is right here with me. When I die I want this to go with me. Thank you so very much." With that comment, I note tears in Colleen's eyes.

But at the very next visit, Colleen meets me at the door, "Maybe that stone wasn't such a good idea. She's lost it several times. We usually can find it, but last night she panicked and nearly fell out of bed reaching over the rails. I heard her crying and got there here just as she stretched for it. I don't think she knows how far it is to the floor."

The hospice aide becomes a heroine by sewing a pouch with a neck strap on it so the stone won't get lost. Carol is now available to Helen at any time.

Several visits later, Colleen is in distress, "She's having hallucinations. She thinks the police are coming in and shooting at her. It took a long time to convince her it was a dream. Could the medication be causing this? Can you give her something for the hallucinations?"

People often see images of their mother or father but I've never heard of them seeing police coming after them, so I quiz Helen about the things she'd seen. There is no mention of loved ones talking to her. I know if anyone would be seeing angels it would be Helen. I note that the television set is less than a foot from the end of her bed.

"Yes," Colleen echoes in with my thoughts as she sees me looking at it, "There was a cop show on, and we were watching it when she drifted off to sleep."

"You don't happen to have a CD player, do you? And some of your mother's favorite music?" I ask. "It's better to use music in place of drugs if it will work—gunshots are pretty hard to drift off to sleep with. In fact, I have a wonderful CD I'll bring the next time I come."

"Oh we have a CD player. Helen's granddaughter, Ellie brought the CD of *"Angels in Training"* followed by *"Calling All Angels."* She puts them in the repeat mode. Helen goes to sleep with pleasant music instead of television noise.

The next time I visit Ellie's there, holding Helen's hands and laughing with her. "You know, my Grandma taught us so much about love. She's always there for us, no matter what's going on."

Helen is smiling at Ellie as she whispers, "I've always loved you, Ellie."

Looking into Helen's eyes, I see that her irises have a gray ring around them—a sign that death is imminent. As I smile at their stories of love, laughter and peace, I know that this woman is nearing her last breath. I have brought a CD titled *"Graceful Passages"* to be played. Helen comments on how much she loves the music.

Colleen walks me to my car and questions how much longer her mother will live. I reply, "I don't have a glass ball to predict her death, but I think it will be very soon. Maybe in the next couple of days, maybe longer. No one can give you that answer, for sure."

"I just don't want her to suffer any longer than she has to," she replies as she hugs me good bye.

Then, as though it was planned, Helen dies the next day.

Later, Colleen calls to remind me that I had promised her mother I'd come to her memorial service. She asks if she can use the CD I'd lent them at the service. I say of course she can. I promise to try to attend the service.

Attending funerals for those I've midwifed until death is very rare for me. I feel that when death happens I pass a baton of compassion to the official bereavement team. Maybe this is a coping skill I've developed because I must immediately be present for another family.

The next Wednesday at the exact time I would have been visiting Helen in her home, I'm walking through the line to pay my respects. The music playing is the music which replaced the police story two weeks before. The angel stone named Carol is in her hand as she lies in the casket.

Author's notes: Chapter 14
The Angel Stone

Note 1: The ambiance in the room of the dying person is important. I had the television turned off and the CD player on when Helen was going to sleep to give her a more peaceful environment. I also moved the bed so she could look out the window and enjoy the birds.

Note 2: Colleen participated in bereavement counseling after her mother died. This is provided by the agency at no charge. The staff who worked with Helen was given time off to go to her funeral if they wanted to.

Note 3: It was my intention for Helen to continue enjoying her Bingo times as long as she could, so providing her with the small oxygen tanks added to her quality of life.

Note 4: I went to the annual bereavement ceremony to honor Helen's life. The agency allots time during the coordination of care conferences to honor the lives of those for whom hospice provided care. The annual ceremony is another time to honor the lives of hospice patients.

She Deserted Me

Why is she leaving me now
Doesn't she remember that she promised
I'd leave first
We made this agreement
I can't live without her
She knows that
Why did she have to go
Where is God's justice
Doesn't he know
How much I need her
Doesn't he care about me
Why didn't I die first
I'll be a hollow shell
No
I won't let her go
She can't die

While driving to my next assigned visit, I hear an internal voice urging me to stop at a local flower shop and buy a rose for Jo. Unable to dismiss the insistent thought, I pull into Jean's Flowers and pick a yellow rose. It is a single stem ending with a perfectly formed opening bud. As the clerk wraps it, I smile wondering why I'm doing this.

I would go broke quickly if I bought one of these for each hospice client I see, so why would I make an exception for her?

Arriving at her home, Jo is delighted to see me and smiles as she accepts the rose. "I'll bet you didn't know I was a Rose Festival Queen sixty-five years ago. A yellow rose was named after me," she exclaims. "Just last week, my court sent me a bouquet of long-stemmed yellow roses." I silently thank my intuition and smile as Jo touches the bud.

Jo lives with her devoted husband of 60 years and two small poodles. Their home is a very neat and nicely decorated apartment. Hospice has been referred because of her end-stage cardiac condition. She is experiencing significant shortness of breath, swelling of the ankles and lack of energy. It's obvious that she has been a fastidious homemaker with everything in its place and a place for everything. Andy, her husband, is dependent on her directions for any move he makes, checking in with her before he answers questions I have about her health. Jo is sitting there in a cotton duster; her legs are very puffy but her face is beautiful with the smoothness of an actress in an Olay commercial; her hair is neatly coiffed—like she'd just left the beauty parlor. It's easy to see her as a festival queen.

"She weighs herself every day and then calls it in to her cardiologist for him to adjust the medications," Andy says, explaining why the pills are given in a manner different from the directions on the bottle.

"But of late, nothing is helping to take the increased weight off," Jo interrupts him. "I don't think it's doing any good anymore."

Hearing this and watching her struggle to get from her wheelchair to a kitchen chair, I know the reason for the referral to my agency. She is suffering from congestive heart failure. She probably is not going to respond to any prescriptions changes her doctor makes.

Andy speaks anxiously, "You can make her breathe easier, can't you? Her doctor said you were her last chance to be made comfortable. She's been so miserable for such a long time. I try to do everything for her, but she still insists on being in charge."

My job is cut out for me…Now I know why I brought that rose.

Jo and Andy both agree that a hospital bed at some time would be in order since her head could be elevated, easing some of the reported difficulty breathing at night.

"But not quite yet," Andy says, and she nods her head.

"How come I run out of energy so quickly? Jo asks. I can't even go to the bathroom or sit down at the table without being exhausted. Then it takes me forever to get enough strength to do my housework."

"Imagine holding marbles in your open hands," I place my palms together in front of them. "Pretend each of these marbles are units of energy. When you awaken and start to get up into your wheelchair— you're breathing hard—that takes a marble of energy. Now you move to the toilet, which takes another marble—and another to get back to the chair. Then you turn the wheels of the chair to get to the table using another marble or two. Even with the oxygen in place it still takes energy. Your lungs are filling up with fluid, and the heart is very tired and unable to pump as it should. Your kidneys aren't working well, either. So, you're using these marbles," I now close my hands together, "very quickly they're all gone. What do you have left? Remember, you've used up all the units of energy you held in your hand."

Responding with a smile as she looks over at Andy, Jo says, "I guess I understand. My marbles are all gone and I'm exhausted. And you are saying there is nothing that can be done to help? That I can't get more marbles, is that right?"

"What it means," I say, "is that you will get exhausted sooner than you used to when your heart was functioning better. Congestive heart failure means that the muscle is not working well enough to take the extra fluid off the lungs and allow more energy. In other words, your heart is very tired."

"I have a pacemaker. It's actually a pacemaker with a defibrillator. Doesn't that help my heart beat better?"

I explain that the pacemaker helps the heartbeat but doesn't improve the muscle itself. Both Jo and her husband nod. Andy says the doctor had just told them that at their last visit.

Jo lifts her head defiantly. "If these pills aren't going to help me then I'm not taking any more of them. Can I try that morphine you said would help me? Didn't you say it would make breathing easier?"

Andy appears agitated, shifting from one foot to another. "Are you sure you want to take that? Remember what happened to Keith when he took the morphine? He died right after he started taking it. We need to talk to our kids first." Andy looks at me. "Can you talk to our daughter Shelley?"

I nod, inviting them both to sit down. I explain that many people have concerns with using morphine. "I can give very small doses which usually help right away with the breathing. As we go along, I'll explain to Shelley what we're doing. I'll also call your doctor and let him know your request about stopping the meds."

At my next visit Jo's stopped all the meds except for the liquid morphine. She says, "It's amazing how it helps me to catch my breath. You can order the hospital bed now, but I'm going to use it only if I have to."

Then she surprises me the following week by declaring: "I want to go. I'm ready to go home. I had a dream that I was at the beach with my daughter. It was very calm and quiet. Shelley was a little girl. We were playing in the water." She's speaking between short pants of breath. She pauses then gasps, "I want to go now! Help me!"

Because Andy was a retired fire captain, he has advantage of having experienced many deaths in his line of work. For weeks he's been watching her as she's struggled. He stands beside her, supporting every decision she makes. He quietly looks down at his feet feeling his own pain.

111

At Jo's direction, I call her doctor's office to get the order to have the pacemaker turned off. She hears the call as I follow up with the pacemaker representative and announces, "I'm eating no more food. I want to die today."

Andy and Jo realize that neither the pacemaker representative nor I have the power to make death happen like waving a magic wand. Before I leave, Jo says laughingly—perhaps seeking approval, "I want one more cookie before I die."

Shelley is there when the pacemaker is turned off. She is holding her mother's hand and giving the care only a daughter can give. Shelley calls from Jo's home the next day and asks me to make a visit. She has to leave for a short time and says her mom isn't doing well.

I arrive soon after receiving the call and Jo greets me, speaking in short sentences: "I hurt all over. Every place Shelley or Andy touches hurts so bad. Can I have some more morphine?"

After giving her an increased dose, Andy takes me aside. "I had this dream last night," he says. " I know she couldn't have made it to my bed from the hospital bed, but I felt her body spooning with me. She was so close that I felt her skin next to mine! I am okay now because I know she will be in peace. I told her I will be all right."

Andy calls the next day asking me to come right away, "I think she's dying right now."

I need to pick up supplies from the office, and when I stop there the new director asks if she can go with me for this visit. She's not a nurse and doesn't have hands-on-experience with people actively dying. I prepare her by telling Jo's story and what might be ahead for us.

However, I'm not prepared for the death to happen so quickly after we arrive. Jo takes several very slow breaths and then none. Andy is there holding her hand, softly crying. He appears stunned by her final breath, yet I see acceptance in his face. He is consoled by the hospice director as I make the final calls to the daughter, the doctor and the mortuary.

Jo's daughter Shelley calls about three months later. "Dad died in his sleep last night. He couldn't wait to be with her. Thank you for all you did for my parents and for me."

A small tear rolls down my cheek as I sit looking at the telephone receiver still in my hand. They are together again.

Author's notes: Chapter 15
A Rose for a Queen

Note 1: When I visited Jo for the last time, I knew that she was actively dying—meaning that she showed the signs that indicated she would die in a short time. She had increased salivation—mucus in her mouth—increased difficulty breathing—increased pain—and she was sensitive to the slightest touch. I know this phase can last a few minutes, hours or, in rare cases, even days. Sometimes the term frightens loved ones who think death will occur in minutes.

Note 2: I stayed in her home after death to spend time with the family, to discard any leftover narcotics, to call the equipment company, the physician and the funeral home.

Note 3: Jo had a pacemaker which she asked to have turned off. This was not necessary because when death occurs, a pacemaker will not keep a person alive. The pacemaker representative came out to turn it off per Jo's request.

Sacred Regard

You let me in
Because you knew I was safe.
Our hearts connected on a deep level

You let me in
Not by granting my request.
But by allowing your heart to open

You let me in
To share this journey.

Being connected
Is a privilege and a responsibility.
I must walk in your home
As if on holy ground.

May I hold this privilege
With honor and sacred regard.

You let me in
Because you knew I was safe.
Our hearts connected on a deep level

You let me in
Not by granting my request.
But by allowing your heart to open.

I Can't Say It

"I didn't get to do any gambling, even though that was the plan when I left for Vegas with my son Dean," Myrtle says when I go over to see her in the hospital. I have the assignment to meet with her and her daughter-in-law before she's discharged to home. I notice bruises on Myrtle's arms and assume they're from frequent blood draws or IV placements.

"She's had a rough six months," Debbie says. "While they were in Las Vegas, my husband Dean went to pick her up for dinner. When she didn't answer, he got the hotel to open her door. There she was on the floor. She told Dean she thought it was a stroke. She was right, but she had a cardiac arrest in the hospital, and the doctors planned for her to have open heart surgery."

"Yeah, they told me I'd be better than ever and have plenty more time to gamble when I recovered. I wasn't having any fun in there," interrupts Myrtle.

Debbie continues, "Then they decided they needed to first check out her arteries since she had that stroke. They found bad veins or arteries—whatever causes strokes, so they scheduled a neck surgery—endart...or something like that. But before she could have surgery, she developed congestive heart failure, so she couldn't have either surgery. They sent her home on medications."

"I never got to gamble; what a cheat that was," Myrtle chimes in. "I guess that's what I get for being eighty-three and smoking most of my life. I don't want to come back to any hospital, regardless of where it is. Right now, I just want to go home. Right here in Oregon City."

"She's been in and out of the hospital since that time with more congestive heart failure thing. It's been hard on her having her salt restricted and having to take all the pills. She can be cranky sometimes," Debbie says apologetically as a nurse comes in the room.

The nurse looks at us and nods showing us fresh scratches on her forearm. "I was trying to feed her, and she got mad at me, screaming for salt. She was so mad she did this to me." She quickly leaves the room with the empty lunch tray in her hands.

"Mom, why did you do that? You'll get your salt when you get home," Debbie scolds softly.

"I wanted it now—not later." Myrtle scrunches her face and gives the nurse the finger once she's out of the room. "She came back and cut my nails. Can you believe that?"

"I'm sorry, for the nurse and for you, Myrtle," I say starting my introduction to hospice. I explain the advantages of being with the program, and pique Myrtle's interest when I say that she'll never have to come back to a hospital and will be able to eat whatever she wants.

"Once on hospice, you're Queen Myrtle and will get anything you can eat. If you develop difficulty breathing, we'll make you as comfortable as possible," I explain.

Both Debbie and Myrtle express a desire to have hospice come to Myrtle's home.

Two days later, I enter Myrtle's bedroom and find her unable to respond in a cogent fashion. Dean and Debbie are close by. They're staying in Myrtle's home to provide care.

"She's been hallucinating," Dean states. "She says her mother is right there beside her. She was mad at us for not seeing her. I guess she's seeing people like that other nurse said she might."

Dean's face has worry lines when he says, "Once before, she got so short of breath we had to stop at a hospital on the way to the doctor's office. How can we stop that from happening again?"

"The difference this time is that you have medicine ordered by the doctor," I explain. "You need only make a call to get help either with a visit or by a nurse giving instructions over the phone. We'll come anytime you need us." Myrtle's breathing is fine now, but I give instructions in case she has problems during the night.

"Sharon, you need to come quickly. Mom's frothing at the mouth. I think she's dying," Dean is on the line the next morning. After giving instructions to treat the breathing difficulty, I head out to Myrtle's home.

When I arrive, I see that she has indeed changed and now is in the phase we call "actively dying" as compared to the slower process of letting go. The pulse increases, the breathing increases and there is often mucus in the mouth, appearing as bubbling or frothing. I use a sponge swab to clean out her mouth.

"Dean, I'm so sorry," I say as gently as possible, "She is very close to death. This is when I encourage families to release their loved one by telling them it is okay to let go. Not that you want them to die, but that you realize it is time for them to go. Many people need that permission from loved ones, especially if they have worries for them or about the family."

"How much longer does she have?" Dean asks anxiously. "I can tell she's close. But I can't say it's okay to let go because I don't want her to die. She said that to my dad and within minutes he was dead. I don't want to be responsible for that. I just can't do it. It's all too much. My wife just left for her mammogram appointment. She's been treated for breast cancer. Should I call her back?"

"Yes," I say, "if she wants to be here for Myrtle's death. I can't say how long it will be, but I can say she will transition soon. Debbie can reschedule her appointment. I know she'll want to be here—to support you and Myrtle." I put a call in for the chaplain knowing Dean will need her, especially if Debbie can't get back in time.

I model swabbing her mouth and wiping the mucus away as I listen to Dean telling stories about his mother and their experiences together. He's becoming calmer and is showing more confidence in caring for her. He is now able to give her permission to let go.

In spite of the behavior I saw in the hospital, Myrtle is obviously a very loved woman and gives selflessly to her family. She has raised a granddaughter who had been a runaway and has given financial and emotional support to Dean as his wife went through her bout with cancer.

"She's a wonderful mother. But, you know, I am sixty-two years old," Dean says in a soft tone, "and until two weeks ago, my mother and I had never told each other of our love. I guess we both assumed it and didn't feel it was necessary to talk about it." He caresses her hand, "I wish I'd started a long time ago because it sure feels good to say it and hear it said by your mother. You see, she said it first and then there was no stopping either of us." Dean turns to Myrtle and says, "Mom, I'm so sorry I didn't tell you earlier. I have appreciated all you did for my family and me. I love you and I will miss you."

Debbie is back. She comes in and throws her arms around her husband. Then she begins to share her stories of love and appreciation with her mother-in-law. "There were times when you frustrated me so much, but you were a second Mom to me. I love you." She leans over and kisses Myrtle's cheek.

With medication, Myrtle's breathing slows down. Appearing more comfortable, she is able to let go and takes her last breath.

Each of us in the room holds our own breath unconsciously and then lets it go with a sigh.

Author's notes: Chapter 16
I Can't Say It.

Note: Dean had trouble saying, "It's okay to go, Mom." I believe that most dying folks need to be told that their family will be alright when they are gone and I wait for that to be said. It is thought of as giving permission for the patient to die. Some people have told me they worry that their loved one will think they want them to die, when really it is a way of saying that the family understands and wants to reassure the patient that the family will be okay.

My friend Paula has just been referred to hospice for stage 4 ovarian cancer with metastases to the heart and colon. I visit her at her home prepared to be present for this phase of her journey. I've brought helpful books and several CDs I have used during my hospice practice.

Paula and I been friends for many years and have worked together in a home care setting. She's recently read the manuscript of stories of my experience as a hospice nurse. She said that through her reading she was able to see another side of me apart from our friendship and our shared work experience. I feel that since she's accepted hospice she'll be interested in what I have to say.

"You don't really think I have time to read these books, do you?" she asked kindly but emphatically. Now mind you, she has already had a year of chemotherapy, radiation and surgery. This time frame has included many emergency admissions to the hospital, blood transfusions and multiple antibiotic infusions. She puts her hospital records on the table for me to see the confirmation of her need for hospice.

"My kids were here this weekend and asked me if I had considered Physician Hastened Death. I told them 'No, not as long as the pain medication could be as effective as I've seen in the patients I've cared for.' They were very open in discussing all this with me even to the point of asking what kind of service I want. But, you know, I've just got too much to do to be bothered with any of that." She waves her hand over the deck toward the railing. "I need to get this painted soon, before the rains come. See what I've planted between driving to town and back for treatments, doctors' appointments and blood draws."

"Aren't you kind of angry? I mean you have two beautiful granddaughters and a toddler grandson living here with you. Don't you want to be there for them as they grow up?" I ask trying to explore her unexpressed feelings.

"Why would I be angry and who would it be against?" She looks intently at me and continues, "I am sad I can't be here to see these girls more since they just moved in, but they'll be with me until I die so I'm lucky that way."

Paula's daughter Kate has chosen to relocate from Oklahoma to spend as much time with her mother as possible. She will provide end-of-life care with help from her brothers and their wives.

"I am fortunate that I have succeeded in my purpose—to get my family close together again," Paula says. "I'm glad my daughter has chosen to stay with me until I die."

I think to myself, *This is the very first time I've dealt with a peer as she enters her hospice phase. This will be a challenging situation for anyone who serves as her hospice nurse.* A part of me is glad I live seventy miles away and will be visiting her as a friend.

Paula shows me what she has been doing: planting, painting and even building a fairy house for her granddaughters.

Kate arrives while Paula is showing me all her accomplishments and says, "How do we stop her? She has more energy than I do. I can't keep up with her and my kids. How are we supposed to slow her down?"

As if to reply with a request, Paula sends me to the hardware store to get more paint for the kids' deck chairs. But I respond to Kate's question first. "Don't even try. Let her do what she wants as long as she can."

Paula interrupts me as she holds up a bright yellow spray paint can lid. "I need a pint in this color. And then we'll go to the casino and have dinner. I try to get to the casino at least twice a week. I'm going to win one of those drawings for a car. Then I'll give it to my kids."

The next time I talk to her, Paula has opted for more chemotherapy in order to give her more time with her grandchildren. "The doctor in Seattle said I didn't qualify for the experimental drugs but suggested I try this type of chemo. I can get it right up the street from here."

One month later, she joins me and my husband for dinner before a Doobie Brothers concert. My husband comments to me later, "She is so peaceful and calm. She looks like an angel. Will she look this good always? If I get cancer, I want to look like her."

And indeed, she is elegantly stunning with the chemo-radiation new hair-style. She appears peaceful and healthy, yet tired from the chemo.

"The only tickets they had left were right in front," she says when we meet her at the lounge. "I wonder if I can get a seat a little farther away from the band because you said they'd be loud. Maybe I can pull the cancer card, and they'll relocate me." I smile knowing she is and will continue to do this her way.

When Christmas comes, I receive a package from her. I call to thank her but get no answer. I imagine she's busy with planning a family reunion. Still, on my way home from a beach weekend, I stop by her home to check on her.

"She's not here. She's in the hospital," her daughter-in-law answers the door. "She had a crisis on Christmas Day after we all left. We didn't want to leave, but she insisted that she'd be okay. But when her pain got unbearable, she asked the neighbor to take her to the local hospital. From there, she was transferred to Corvallis where she is now. I'm sorry no one told you."

When I arrive at the hospital the next day, she is recovering from a surgery to repair the damage done by the chemotherapy and the cancer.

"They put a mesh over a tear in the colon, but I'm getting better," she says, greeting me with her typical positivity. "Take a walk with me and we can talk more. Once I have a bowel movement, I can go home." She talks as I help her to circle the nurses' station. "The last real meal I ate was on Christmas Day with all my family. We had lobster and scallops, and it was oh, so good. I think that last dose of chemo did me in."

"Are you considering hospice when you go home?" I ask gently knowing she had signed off of hospice when she started this last round of treatment.

"No," she replies. "I want to get home. Baby steps, Sharon. My family can take care of me. I just need to poop. Then I'll get home and get better. But, hey, I need to lie down."

As we enter her room, the nurse is there to give an enema which she refuses stating, "I don't want or need that."

A week later as I enter her room the phone rings. I hear Paula say, "Oh, hi, yes, I'm here in the hospital— you were right—wait, I can't hear you." She hands the phone to me. "Here, talk to my sister. These nurses want me for something."

On my last visit, Paula had told me her sister Ellen had refused to take a cruise to Australia with her, fearing she might get real sick and die on it. Paula had said me she wasn't worried, "So what if I die? She can have me cremated there since I'm being burned up anyway."

I explain to Ellen what I know about what was going on and that a peripherally inserted central (PIC) line was being put in to provide an intravenous catheter for medications and fluids since her labs were showing imbalances. And a surgery was being planned to relieve an obstruction (severe constipation). When I return to Paula's room, they've started the procedure so I go down to the cafeteria. Seeing her doctor I approach him about her condition.

He answers my queries with patience. "I'm glad to meet you, but I'm not sure what's going on with Paula. She doesn't seem to want to try to get better. She seems to be hiding from the world. Each time I see her, she has her eyes covered with a washcloth, as if she wants it all to go away. Her condition could be treated with more chemo if she'd only try. Right now, I ask her what she needs and then give it to her."

When I return to her room, Paula's eyes are covered, and the intravenous line is in place. "They're going to give me TPN (total parenteral nutrition-IV solution to replace missing nutrition). I'm not sure I want it." She speaks so softly that I must bend down to hear her.

I respond quickly. "You don't have to have it if you don't want it."

"Well, I do if I want to live," she retorts. "I need to get back home."

Surgery is done and a colostomy placed as the surgeons had anticipated. The colon is too damaged to hold the stitches due to the effects of cancer and chemotherapy.

At my next visit, I find Paula in the bathroom nauseated and in pain. At first she doesn't recognize me and thinks I am a hospital nurse until she gets back into bed and looks up at me.

"Oh, it's you," she says. I look into the eyes of a person who has given up. Her face is wan; her pain is high—8 out of 10 on a 10 scale— and she is miserable.

"I don't want this thing," she exclaims as she touches the colostomy bag. "I told them before I went to surgery, and it's still true." Her oldest son is visiting and asks the nurse for pain medication and something for nausea.

The rest of this visit, I try to understand what she really wants. She speaks sparingly and then only in an unintelligible whisper. I watch as the nurse attempts to get the pain under control with an intravenous dose. The pump has been taken away due to a misunderstanding between the surgeon and the nursing staff. When the patient-controlled device has been restarted, it takes several doses to get the pain under control. The pump is designed so a patient can push a button for comfort—at predetermined intervals to prevent overdosing. If needed the interval can be decreased or the amount delivered increased.

Perhaps she really does want to be free of all of this and medicate herself heavily. I see her spirit leaving unless we can get her out of here and home where her grandkids and family are.

A surgeon enters the room and tells her, "If you want to go home, you're going to have to get up and walk and eat and have the colostomy working."

Turning to me, he explains the outcome of the surgery. I then ask him, "If this were your mother or aunt in this bed what would you expect the course of events to be from here? Do you see success with this surgery or will her bowels continue to be affected downstream from the colostomy hook-up?" I want to know and want Paula to hear what she has to look forward to if she does all the requirements and goes home.

"Yes, I expect her to have more problems, and the bowels will probably continue to tear, but we don't know that," he responds. "But she must be eating before she leaves here."

At that moment I feel committed to getting her home as soon as possible. *If they don't start plans to get her out of here soon, she will die. I can't let that happen to my friend. She needs to be in her home with her grandkids and to see the beach again.*

I call her family and give my evaluation and advise that she could go home under hospice and be with those she loves. Her family understands and starts the action. Her oldest son works for an ambulance company. He gets approval for a transfer from his company and implores the driver to provide a "smooth ride for very precious cargo."

The following weekend when I go to visit, I find that hospice is providing equipment, the pain pump and support. I join Paula and her family on a trip to the beach. Managing a pain pump, an oxygen tank, six kids, seven adults and a beach wheelchair is a challenge. Paula is very weak after being in the hospital for the last six weeks. It's obvious to me that the family will grant her wishes if at all possible. Paula is determined to make it happen so she is agreeable to all suggestions.

She shines as we tuck blankets and coats around her to protect her from the cold spring wind. She smiles as she watches her grandkids cavort energetically and playfully around the sand and rocks. Two people are needed to pull and steady the wheelchair as it is placed into a perfect position for her to watch the waves. Paula is ecstatic, and we are as well.

At one point her son asks, "So, what else is on your bucket list, Mom? You've skydived and saw Chiluly's glass museum. What else can we do for you?"

"I want to sail," she quickly responds.

"On a sailboat or using your remote controlled sailboat?"

"Both," she answers. "Can I have that peanut butter sandwich you promised me, Kate? And I want an ice cream cone before we go home."

On return, Paula insists on trying to walk into the house. "I'm going to get better. Just watch and see."

Paula has endeared herself to many loving people so now, when needed, volunteers come forward to provide night coverage so the family can rest.

"Isn't it amazing how well I'm provided for?" Paula asks me at my next visit. "I mean I was able to get this home before my other house in Portland went into foreclosure. And I got everything done I wanted to before I got too sick. I even had my gas fireplace done while I was in the hospital so it would be ready when I came home. And now I have my two beautiful granddaughters here; my other grandkids come to see me. I am so grateful. My kids did well to get me out of that place. I was going crazy there. They would have killed me with medications if I stayed. They tried to give me a medication that I remember refusing to give a patient when I was working as a nurse because of its side effects. But I said no, I won't take it. We've seen lots of changes over the years, haven't we, Sharon?"

I nod and take the opportunity to read a chapter from the book titled *Heaven Really Does Exist* lying at her bedside.

"It's a great book," she explains before I start, "it's about a little boy who tells his mother and father about his visit to heaven weeks after being critically ill and the surgery which saved him."

When I finish the chapter, she says, "Yes, I know it exists—heaven, that is. I will walk off this earth onto a cloud. Then Jesus will meet me and take me to meet God."

The hospice aide arrives to bathe her so I go with Kate to another room. As I leave, I hear Paula say, "There's a first time for everything. This will be the first time I've been bathed in front of a gas fireplace. You know, my sons just finished it."

When I return after the bath, she asks, "What were you two doing in there? There was a lot of laughter! I'm sure glad you came to see us."

I read her favorite psalm to her—the twenty-third and leave when she falls asleep.

A week has passed when the phone rings. "Can you come?" Kate asks. "It's very hard. Mom's not talking, and she's barely eating. I thought I was doing well, but right now I feel like I'm losing it."

When I arrive I see a body with little or no response. Paula's cheeks are sunken, her color pale, her eyes are closed with a washcloth over them. A neighbor is there to watch while Kate and her aunt are running errands.

Not knowing my experience as a hospice nurse, he demonstrates how to give her water—by holding a finger over the tip of a straw and then dropping it on her mouth. I pick up the sponge stick, moisten it and put in her mouth to suck on. Paula looks up at me and smiles. Her head is arched back. She is coughing. I lift her so she can cough more effectively. *Using the straw method of giving fluids is often the cause of pneumonia so the sponge is the ideal way—that way she will only swallow after she's sucked. Dropping the fluid in can result in it going down the windpipe.*

Taking a chair next to her bed, I read a poem to Paula about being grateful and trusting any unfinished business will be carried on by those still here. Immediately she opens her eyes and says the names of her three children as if designating them to complete her tasks. As I read on there is a statement about letting go and once more she opens her eyes. She puts her hands up to her face and says, "This is so weird! Am I still here?" Then she pats her face and continues, "Am I really here?" I hear disbelief in her voice, like she is sure she is not here but elsewhere.

"Yes, Paula dear, you are still here but not for long. I love you. I'm going to miss you terribly, but I know you must go."

Kate returns home with her daughter, and they both speak to Paula with no apparent response from her.

I show Paula's granddaughter a kids' book I've found. It's about a nymph becoming a dragonfly and accepting the transition from one form to another. Essentially it is a book about accepting death. These girls certainly need all the help they can get for they are about to lose this woman who is very dear to them. As I read, I note that Paula, her daughter and granddaughter are attentive to the story. Paula's head is turned toward me as Kate, Cahleigh and I are sitting on the bed.

Now as Paula listens to the story of the dragonfly, she appears to wait until I'm finished before she starts coughing yet again. Kate and I lift her up as she attempts to clear her throat. I note her discomfort and share that with Kate.

"The hospice doctor said we could increase the medications, but I'm afraid to do it. Do you think we should?" She asks.

"If you feel she is suffering you should discuss that with your nurse. But yes, I see her uncomfortable and restless as she is fidgeting in the bed," I reply, knowing her regular hospice nurse is off today. However, a substitute is due any time, and Kate can check with her.

I am especially touched when Kate relates what her mom told her when she was still alert enough to talk. "She tells me of being in this beautiful field with a man in the distance. There was a locked gate, and she held the key. When I asked her if the man was my dad, she nodded.

When I asked her why she didn't use the key, she replied, 'Then I would be gone.' I told her it was perfect for her to be with Dad. I said we would miss her, but I knew she had to go."

Laughingly, Kate told me about the last weekend. "Mom wanted to have a special celebration with the family. I think she wanted to soften the children's fears of her dying. Mom got all dressed up with blue nail polish and a cute pixie cut hairstyle. She even got a massage. My brothers pushed the hospital bed out on the deck. She led a ceremony about her going to be with Jesus. We released Chinese lighted balloons into the night. It was beautiful." Tears are now rolling down both our cheeks.

Three days later I hear the message Kate left on the answering machine. "Mom died this morning at 10:30. The family was here over the weekend telling her how much she was loved. The girls were at school. It's over, now."

Four weeks have passed and I stand before an altar displaying Paula's nursing school graduation picture. Looking into her eyes I am amazed to feel the energy coming over me. Here I am looking at her while seeing myself in that picture as well. For, you see, we graduated at the same time, wore our hair in the same style and even had the same nursing caps. Now I look at the words we shared as a motto of life: LIVE WELL, LAUGH OFTEN, LOVE MUCH. Paula had written these words on many gifts to me and to others—even to the point of having them printed on the teabags at the reception. Now these words are on little tiles, ensconced in a tray of sand circled with sea shells. For a brief moment, I see a bigger picture of life and then I see myself as the one being grieved. I think of how much I've learned as I traveled this path of midwifeing the soul and body into death. I recall a quote and now know the truth of it:

**"While I thought that I was learning how to live,
I have been learning how to die**."
Leonardo da Vinci

Goodbye my Dear Friend
Goodbye and Thank You.

Author's notes: Chapter 17
Good-by to a Friend.

Note: Paula chose to go off hospice for more chemotherapy. It is possible to go off and then sign back on hospice if the treatment is ineffective, if it has too many side effects or it is just refused.

=

DEATH: Mine and Yours

How will death come?
Will it be quick and painless
Or drawn out and full of suffering?

Will family surround me
As I breathe my last breath?
Will Love and Forgiveness be at my bedside?
Will I die with my eyes wide open?

Perhaps I will hold an audience
Inviting those I've loved
To be there to hold my hand?
Or maybe I will want to be alone?

Will I be conscious
Knowing of death as passing thru a door
Excited at my next adventure
Accepting Heaven as the perfect moment?

Death is our lifetime uninvited guest
Beside us since birth
Closer than our breath
As disregarded as our shadow.

THE LADY WHO KNEW WHAT SHE WANTED

"I don't want to be here any longer," Bea tells me as we sit in her apartment with the spring sunlight streaming in. "I've been here ninety-four years. There's nothing left for me to do, and I'm never going to be what I was in my past."

Bea suffers from a brittle form of diabetes. Her blood sugars vacillate from hypoglycemic to hyperglycemic quickly and are difficult to control. She has high blood pressure and residual damage from a stroke several years ago.

"I'm not sure what you mean, Bea," I reply. "You say you're tired of living. I met your daughter and see pictures of your grandchildren. Your family seems to be close to you—I'm sure they want to support you as much as possible."

"I know," she says, "but there's no fun in living anymore. I've had a good life. I've gone fishing, hiking, skiing. I have friends—but I no longer can carry on a conversation. I know what I want to say, but I can't get the right word out—it just won't come out the way I want it to. I can't see, and I don't hear well. I don't want to be a burden. I'm just through with life."

With the help of the assisted living facility staff, Bea and her seventy-four-year-old daughter have been able to manage checking her blood sugar and monitoring food intake. But Bea is tired of all the effort she requires.

She has asked for hospice to become involved so she can be allowed to die. My task is to listen and to problem solve with her and her daughter, Donna. I am to be as present as possible should another event occur, such as her recent hospitalization for out-of-control-diabetes.

"I never want to go back to the hospital," she states matter-of-factly. "Why can't you medical people understand?"

135

"I do understand. I'll call your doctor and see what he thinks of following your wishes and discontinuing some of your medication, as you request. We'll have trouble eliminating the insulin, but the blood pressure meds might be slowly decreased until you're not taking any. You know of course, the effects of untreated high blood pressure—a stroke can happen. If the doctor approves and makes the changes, I'll talk with the facility manager since we'll need to be prepared in case something happens after the medication changes. They can't provide staff around the clock so if something happened they'd need to call 911 and send you to the hospital," I explain.

"Well," she counters, "the doctor and I both signed that form you gave us on your first visit. It said I didn't want any extra measures given to me if I required urgent care."

My next act is to call her daughter. She approves of her mother doing things her way, but is sad to hear of Bea's distress.

"I love my mom. I know she's been unhappy and thinks hospice can help her," she says. "She's tired of living. Do you think the doctor will agree to take away those pills?" She pauses. "I don't want her thinking she's a burden. I only live ten minutes away and love to visit her—but that's not enough. She doesn't want to go to the cafeteria because she can't hear and can't carry on a conversation with other people. She used to be so active—always doing something."

I tell her I understand her feelings and that we'll talk again soon.

After leaving Bea's apartment, I call the doctor's office then stop at the manager's office to clarify the coming changes. Sitting behind a big desk is a big man with a gentle demeanor and a smile.

"That's good that you talked to her doctor. But if she has a stroke or goes into a diabetic coma, we'll still have to call 911. That's our policy. We can't do it any other way. Our staff is trained to respond to a medical emergency, and I can't make an exception for a hospice patient. What if a maid went into her room and she was unresponsive? I'm sorry, but she'll have to move to another place if that's what she wants."

"If that's your policy, I'll have to go back to the drawing board." I write the order to decrease Bea's medications and return to my office to talk to our medical director.

There is a hospice-care facility available for end-of-life care like this, but several doctors need to review her case and determine her eligibility for residence. She must also have a psychological consult to rule out depression.

"Well," Bea tells me at my next visit, "I told that man that I was not depressed, just tired of living. How can he sit there in front of me and tell me I'm depressed? I'm done with this life. I can never go back to the way I was and that's it. Oh, they can keep me alive for another ten years, but it's not worth it to me. I told him that it's my life, and I want it to be my death."

After the psychologist reports to the doctors that she isn't depressed, I visit Bea again, "We can move you to a hospital-like setting where your blood pressure will be monitored and medications tapered down until they can be stopped. Your insulin can also be stopped."

"How will that work?" Bea asks. " But I'm glad to hear that somebody's going to listen to me. So when can I go?"

"Soon. The medical director of the facility will be in charge of the orders. He or she will make the changes in those meds and insure your comfort throughout. The staff here is familiar with hospice patients and will be delighted to have you there. Do want some time to tell your friends here and your family?" I ask.

"No," she says, and I notice her difficulties as she struggles for the right words. "It's nobody's business but mine. I'll tell my daughter, Donna, and you tell the manager here that I'm moving—he needs no other explanation."

I'm asked to give a report to the staff after her transfer is complete. "Yes," I say to a roomful of doctors and nurses, "she wants to die and feels no one wants to let her stop her medications." I explain the policies of the assisted-care facility she came from.

"Are you telling us that Bea is having existential suffering? Is this what this is all about?" The medical director asks, appearing to be looking right through me. At that moment I empathize with the nurses sitting around the table. They will be working with Bea as the medications are withheld, knowing her blood sugars will rise quickly as the insulin is decreased. She will suffer high blood sugars much sooner than have a stroke from high blood pressure.

"Yes," I replied. "I believe that she is suffering and can find no release from that."

Bea remains at the hospice facility. When I visit her, she beams with a smile that thanks me for facilitating her death without physical or emotional suffering. Bea's family is present daily to see her and even bring her Godiva chocolates. She only eats one or two pieces, but she is very pleased to have those.

Bea becomes very sleepy. She eats less but has no pain and appears happy.

Three weeks later she dies surrounded by family.

Author's Notes: Chapter 18
The Lady Who Knew What She Wanted

Note 1: It seemed that Bea had lost all sense of meaning to her life. For her to continue would have meant suffering. She felt she was complete and expressed this by asking to be allowed to die. Here is an example of existential suffering—a pain that is of a spiritual not a physical nature.

Note 2: The facility Bea was admitted to and died in is used for immediate end-of-life care or for pain care that cannot be handled in the home setting.

BUTTERFLY SOCKS

It bothers me when I can't find my butterfly socks on a cool morning. Frustrated, I pull everything out until I find one of the two pairs I had. Silly though it may seem, I grieve for my mother who died eight years ago. I cry for a brief moment as I hold the gift I gave her only days before her death. A rush of emotions overwhelms me as those two months before her death flood my memory.

Mom and I are shopping at Fred Meyer's. She delights in finding things she's never seen before.

"What is it?" She asks as she picks up an exotic fruit or vegetable. "I've never tasted anything looking like this. Can we get one?" Sometimes a shopping trip takes twice or even three times longer than it would have in the past and we end up with some pretty bizarre items like cactus and cardamom seeds.

Today as we pass a rack of clothes, I comment on the multi-colored butterflies on a display of socks.

"Oh, I love them," she exclaims. "I've never worn socks with butter-flies on them."

"Let's buy a pair for you and one for me," I reply putting two pairs in the basket.

Mom smiles much like a child with a new toy. "Thank you, but you don't need to do that."

My mother has had a rough eighty-two years, but now she's settled into a comfortable life in an assisted retirement apartment building. My sister and I moved her here after she began to show signs of dementia with some delusions— and overall inability to care for herself. And she was three hundred miles away from us. She accepted her new life with hesitancy, guarded in her enthusiasm but willing to give up her old life to be near us.

After a rough start, our relationship began to change—for the better. She used to say, "You sound too much like a nurse asking all these questions." I realize now that she wants a daughter, not a clinician, and she responds to my love without the "nurse-talk." I used to quiz her about her blood tests, medications and appetite. Not anymore!

I make an appointment with a geriatric specialist because I am concerned about her mental status. At her first appointment, she asks for that pink form, "You know the one I mean, Doctor. The one that says you'll let me go if there's nothing that will help me."

Doctor Patty Newton looks at her quizzically, "Oh, you mean the POLST form? The Physician's Order for Life Sustaining Treatment—is that what you want?"

"Yes, I want you to sign one so I can have it in my refrigerator," Mom explains. "That's where the retirement place I live in keeps things like that—in a tube in the refrigerator. I'm supposed to put a list of my medicines there along with my family phone numbers. Sharon told me about all this stuff—she's a hospice nurse, you know," she finishes with a proud look on her face.

Over the years I had felt disapproval and disappointment from my parents, especially my mother, but not today. Mom had expressed her displeasure in my life choices, like me not going into "God's work," something I said I would at age seventeen. She also didn't like my divorce or my second husband. I really got on her bad side when I started drinking beer, not going to church and spending my free time running and playing tennis. She made disparaging remarks every chance she could.

"You, of all people, should know better than to do this or that," she'd say, whatever the complaint *du jour* was, whether it was buying new tennis shoes while my daughter wore her chosen grunge clothes or keeping "too clean of a house" for her tastes.

But today I feel my mother is proud of me. I haven't prompted her at all, and I'm delightfully surprised that she expresses her needs.

"I can certainly sign that paper, but why do you feel you need it?" The doctor asks her, looking over at me. "I mean, I don't see that you have any real physical problems right now. What are your reasons?"

"Well, first thing is, I'm old. Second thing is, God and I have an arrangement. He and I are in agreement that I will die before I become dependent, before I can't recognize my children and before I have cancer," Mom explains to her new primary doctor. The doctor looks at me and flashes a big smile. *Did I say she couldn't take care of herself?*

Mom continues, "I want to make sure no one stops me from dying in God's time—I read too much about people on machines when they should be able to join Jesus."

"OK, I'll get the POLST form and go over it with you next time you see me. But first, I'm going to give you five items to remember. Then I'll ask you to repeat them later," Dr. Newton remembers the information I'd told her prior to our visit. I'd mentioned her memory loss and occasional confusion.

At our next appointment, the doctor has the results of blood tests and the pink form. She reviews the choices with Mom.

" Antibiotics?"

" No".

"Resuscitation?"

"No.

"Comfort measures only?"

"Yes."

After signing it, the doctor hands it to her. "Now, you can put it in that tube you mentioned last week. Does the manager of the building really want it in the fridge?"

Mom nods. "That way the ambulance drivers know where to look for it. I know it sounds weird, doesn't it?"

"Mrs. White," Dr. Newton says, "your memory is definitely worsening, according to your family and by the results of your memory test. I do have some medications that might help that if you'd like to give them a try."

My mother agrees, but then after one week's trial of Aricept and Namenda, she tells me and my sister, "These things make me feel drugged, and I feel like I'm losing it! If you two keep meddling in my life, I will kill myself."

Understanding this is an idle threat, we are still shocked and frustrated at being put in our places. So we encourage her to tell her doctor she wants to stop the pills, a call she makes without any hesitation. The doctor agrees that it is her choice.

Mom adjusts to being in a facility. Over time, my sister and I assume more and more of her care. We bring her laundry home and take her shopping. When I bring her to my home for the day or a weekend, she asks me about my hospice patients and how people respond to hospice services.

One day she says, "I'm glad you are a hospice nurse. I know that I've lived long enough, and I'm ready to go to heaven. When something happens to me, I want you to be the one to find me. Your sister isn't prepared like you are. I plan to die in my sleep, just not wake up some morning. I don't want her coming into my apartment and finding my body. I won't be here for my next birthday—eighty-three years is too long to live. I have nothing left to do. It's time I go."

"Mom, it'd be nice if it happens the way you want," I say gently. "Many people say they wish to die in their sleep. They also say they don't want cancer or dementia, but I don't believe we have any control over those things. If, indeed you do, I'd like to know how to do it."

"It's my connection with God. You will have to do that on your own. I can't do it for you," she replies.

Mom has a deep spiritual belief. She's always reading her Bible and used to teach Bible study groups. Even as a toddler, I was hauled to church at least three times a week. In retrospect I wonder why I was the one to go while my siblings were allowed to stay home. I remember how Mom was always helping the elderly—taking them to medical appointments, to church or shopping. I think I owe my love of the older population to her.

Maybe Mom feels she's finished her assigned task—no more older ladies to transport hither and yon, no more Bible Study classes, no more church services to attend or potluck dinner dishes to make. Now, she sits and thinks about her life.

One day she says, "I guess I have to learn to live before I can die. I can't let any opportunity pass since I know my time is limited. I'm not having another birthday."

"I don't understand why my sons aren't calling me back. I've called them both and left messages. I'd like to see them before I die," she says sadly

I'm disappointed by my brothers' lack of interest in our mother's health. I call my older brother.

"So what," my older brother says when I tell him of her decline, "She's an old woman, and she's gonna die soon—what do you want me to do about it? I'm not coming up to visit her, and I'm not calling her," click. No goodbye or thanks for calling.

"I don't understand why my sons aren't calling me back. I've called them both and left messages. I'd like to see them before I die," she says sadly.

The subject of my little brother comes up again on a later visit. "I need to talk to you about your little brother. He won't answer me, even when I leave a message on his phone." Mom settles into a recliner. "I've never told anybody—but I really didn't want him and I know I've been holding that against him all his life." She proceeds to tell the story of her sadness of leaving downtown Santa Monica to come to start a new life with her family of five—three kids under five years old living in a tent in the middle of winter in rainy southern Oregon.

"I need to get this off my chest. I didn't want another kid—I wasn't able to care for the ones I had, but your father forced me to have my fourth. I wasn't feeling good. It was right after I had my teeth pulled," she stops to take a big breath.

I remember her telling me that because she had a single cavity, Dad had insisted on having all her teeth pulled, because forty miles was too far to go to the dentist.

Continuing but now sobbing she says, "He said he'd leave me if I didn't give in. What was I to do?" She looks up at me as I hold her close.

"I'm sorry. I shouldn't have said this. Now you'll think poorly of your father." More tears—*my mother is so very fragile*—I think as I hug her.

145

"Mom," I reassure her. "Mom, Dad's been dead for twelve years. I'm not going to think any less of him with your comments. You don't need to keep this inside you. You aren't responsible for what I think of him. Don't worry about it." I feel the smallness of her body as she pulls away from my arms.

"I never wanted your brother and I tried to make it up to him by protecting him," she says looking at me for acceptance. Receiving a nod, she proceeds, "Forgive me for being angry at you that summer day. I remember you wanted to call the police on him. I should have let you. Maybe things would have been better."

How well I remember that moment. I was sixteen and Larry was thirteen when he threw Mom on the floor and pinned her down with his knee—he was angry that the hot chocolate she made was so hot it burned his tongue. Mom told me to go away and never get between her and him again.

"I know now how worried you were for me. I'm so very sorry for all that I did. I could never tell anyone this, not even a doctor or a minister. I do wish I could talk to your brother and explain things. I should never have had him, but I did. And I couldn't deal with him wisely." She wipes her tears on her sleeve.

She sits in the big recliner looking like her life force has been sucked out of her, but finishes with, "I'm so glad to be able to tell someone this—it's been so painfully long! Can you take me home now? I'm very tired."

On the drive to her assisted-living apartment, she speaks softly about her death. "God and I have this agreement; I'm going to die one night and just not wake up. I've learned how to live now, so I can go."

Her peaceful confidence envelops me. I think of my dad and the news that he had forced himself on his wife at a very vulnerable time. I knew she had no birth control, and raising four kids without running water or electricity must have been so hard. I now feel more compassion for my brother.

When I stop at Mom's several weeks later, I see her laying her binoculars aside. "I was using these to see you as you come down the Fremont Bridge. I've been thinking about you and your sister....She's going to need to forgive if she ever expects to be forgiven. She can't hold grudges against her boys like she's doing."

That's my Mom. Always trying to solve everybody's problems. I smiled and said nothing.

Shortly after this, I have a dream about my mother's death. I share this with Anne, a social worker friend the next day.

"You were in it, Anne. You were helping solve the problem—of getting my mother's body home when she died on a trip to San Francisco. In the dream you were in San Francisco ,and you found the casket that I used to transport her to Portland," I explain to her. "I don't know what it means, but thanks for the help."

Four days later during a staff meeting, I hear an overhead announcement for an outside call for me. It interrupts a meeting where we acknowledge and remember patients who have died in the last two weeks. A mixed bag of emotions is expressed from tears to laughter and thankfulness that this particular one has finally died.

"Yes, this is Sharon White," I answer the call on line 1. "Yes, Bessie is my mother. You did what? You just found her dead!" I scream into the phone. "Yes, I'll be right there."

Suddenly, my well-organized world totally falls apart. A large hole opens, and I am swallowed up. After years of being a nurse, of being aware of my mother's aging process, years of comforting and caring for many patients and their families—I am now facing death, and I am totally lost. I'm crying so hard and so loud that I can't answer the questions from those who surround me wanting to know what's wrong.

"She died. She just died. Just like that," I blurt out between sobs.

"Who died? Who was it? Sharon, answer me." My friend Anne from the next cubicle is hugging me. "Was it Ruth? Which patient died, Sharon?"

The receptionist answers when I can't, "It's her mother. I just took the call from Marshall Union Manor."

I wilt into the arms of those who've just shared their grief for the deaths of patients we've been caring for. The world stops turning for this brief moment in time. Then, almost as quickly, my training kicks into action, and I start thinking of all the patients I am scheduled to see today, of all the calls to doctors' offices and of the medications I must pick up before my visit. Just before I sink into debilitating thoughts, I transfer my duties my supervisor. I can't think beyond this moment.

"Whom can I call for you? Can I reach your husband?" The chaplain is there at my side writing down names of contact people.

"My husband has just returned from a three month job out of town. My sister has gone to Coos Bay; I don't know where she can be reached. I have to go—the facility is expecting me." I'm trying to tie the loose ends of my planned day

When I reach my husband, I sob the news. "I need you to look on my desk—the right side. Mom and I just finished making the final arrangements for her burial last week. There's a folder there. Please bring it to me." *I'm so grateful I insisted she finalize her wishes. She had hesitated over burial or cremation, finally choosing burial to please her estranged sons.*

"You aren't going by yourself, are you?" Anne asks. "You can't do that, I'm coming with you. You just told me about your dream and I was in that dream, so I'm coming with you—I intend to complete my part of it."

During the half mile drive to Mom's apartment, I think about the dream. Anne had been there to help me, so now I'm grateful she will be with me. My thoughts are running as fast as my tears are flowing.

"Kory will take you up to the apartment," the secretary says, handing me a tissue to wipe my tears. Kory is the manager and has spent time talking to Mom.

"When she didn't pick up her paper as she does every morning," Kory says as he pushes the button for the elevator, "her neighbor called the maintenance man to check on her—that's when he found her on her sofa. I'm so very sorry." He opens the door and turns to leave. "Let me know if I can do anything for you. Bessie was a very nice person. I'll miss chatting with her." He pulls the door shut.

Here I am, alone with death.

I've been here many times before, but never with my own mother. Tears cascading down my cheeks, I lean over to kiss her. She's sitting up with her Bible on her left side. Her glasses are a bit askew and she's cold.... oh so very cold. Fully dressed, reading her Bible, she has died, just like she said she would. Her eyes are wide open, no trace of fear or pain to be seen. *She should be answering me, a part of me thinks.*

The door opens. Anne comes in me and hugs me. My husband follows and holds me as I cry. We take her glasses off and lay her stiffened body on her sofa. I close her eyes, giving another kiss to this woman who gave me life.

Suddenly the practices and duties of my hospice training are recalled as if from rote memory, and my hospice skills take over. I make calls to my sister, to the doctor's office and to the mortuary. As a social worker, Anne knows this routine very well. She takes as many of the tasks as she can such as looking up numbers, calling to see which local mortuary handles the transportation of caskets to Coos Bay from Portland.

A knock on the door brings me back to this moment. "It's the mortuary," a voice calls out. The dreaded finality is in front of me. A gurney is lowered to couch level, the quilt removed and the body bag unzipped the length of the stretcher. I assist transferring the precious cargo which housed my mother's spirit to the gurney, place the quilt on her and zip up the bag to her chin. A final kiss and I close the remaining inches of the zipper, pulling the quilt over her body. I then crumble to my knees in my husband's arms.

Good-bye.

Thank You.

Thank you for preparing me for all the synchronistic events surrounding your death. Your timing was impeccable. You waited until my husband had returned from out of town. You didn't have a painful nor confused death. You didn't have cancer. You fell asleep...just like you promised. You had the opportunity to say a final goodbye, expressing your love to my sister the night before your death.

All my siblings attended Mom's funeral. My brothers were there to tell her how much they loved her and would miss her.

So, today, when I put those socks on, I send a message of gratitude to the woman who "never had socks with butterflies on them." Maybe I'll never throw them away!

149

Author's notes: Chapter 19

Butterfly Socks

Note 1: In Oregon, the *Physician's Order for Life Sustaining Treatment* is printed on bright pink paper. (It is state-specific.) Considered a doctor's order as its name implies, emergency personnel are obligated to follow it when they are called. It outlines choices for hospice patients—and whether or not they wish aggressive intervention or comfort measures.

PART FIVE

Non-Judgmental Care

I Will Not Leave My Home

Ruth is ninety-one, living alone and bedridden. She has fired several nurses because they've tried to tell her she needed to be able to move in an emergency in order to be safe.

"I don't care if there is a fire—I will burn with my home. I'm going to be cremated anyway," she informed the first nurse she sent packing.

The second one was dismissed because she wanted to order more equipment than Ruth thought she needed. A male nurse was told to not come back because she dislikes men.

"Pomeroy is my guard cat, and he doesn't like men," Ruth explains as I take on the challenge to work with her. "I'm not trying to be difficult. It's just that I've lived in this neighborhood for 65 years and everybody looks in on me. I have a friend who comes in every day before she goes to work at Oaks Park."

"What do you do when you need to urinate?" I ask simply, knowing I could be dismissed if my questions are too intrusive.

"Oh, I just hold it until she gets here; she comes every morning."

I realize that if I am to be accepted here until her death, I must give up requirements or conditions. Entering Ruth's world, I must be willing to let her die as she wishes and let her remain in her home as long as she is safe and alert.

"I like you," Ruth says after the second visit. "You can keep coming to see me. My niece will be here next week. Will you come and meet her?" She asks tentatively.

Meredith shakes my hand and tells me that she is confident her aunt is okay. "Her friend and really the entire neighborhood keep their eyes on her. She's a damn feisty and independent woman. My mom, her sister, was just like her. I won't hold anyone responsible if something happens, like if she falls out of bed and has to lie there until someone finds her."

She gives her aunt a kiss. Teasing, Meredith asks, "How many men has Pomeroy chased away, Auntie?" She turns to me and asks, "Has she told you about him?" We all laugh as I relate how Pomeroy is the reason I am here. "Ruth's family is me and two cousins. We've learned to leave you alone haven't we, Aunt Ruth? I live in Bend and come over twice a month. Are you doing okay, Auntie?"

"Yes," Ruth replies with a twinkle in her eye, "except I'm dying." Her frail body shakes with laughter.

Meredith stays only long enough to give support and check on the food supply. "Call me if you have any concerns," she says as she gets into her SUV and drives away.

"Can you come quickly?" Ruth's friend is calling me two days later. "She's struggling to breathe, and she hasn't peed for two days now."

"I'll be right there," I say and put aside all other calls.

As soon as I arrive, I give Ruth a dose of morphine. Fortunately, this is routinely delivered to hospice patients as soon as possible since a large percentage of those who come on board develop a crisis within a few days.

Twenty minutes after I give her the morphine, Ruth's breathing improves slightly. I catheterize her for a large amount of urine. Then quickly, within six minutes, she takes her last breath.

Indeed, Ruth met death her way.

Author's notes: Chapter 20
I Will Not Leave My Home

Note 1: Ruth's wishes were to be respected as long as she was safe. I deemed it appropriate to allow her to remain in her home since her niece, her power of attorney, had requested that she stay.

Note 2: I have seen other patients react and let go as Ruth did when I gave her the morphine.

I haven't been in John's home for ten minutes when he takes a card from his wallet and holds it out. It is a membership card for the Mormon Church. "This is my guarantee that I'm going to heaven," he says, waving the card, "so I don't have to worry about dying. When we're given this, we know heaven is our destination. Pretty good, isn't it?" He continues after putting the card away.

"I prayed for God to take my pain away, and He did. Now I don't have any. I think I'll be fine and probably I won't need you folks. My doctor said there's nothing more he can do but that you folks will be able to help me to the end. I'm more concerned about my brother, Sam, than I am about myself. You see, he's older and I've always taken care of him. Before, the pain was so bad that I thought I wouldn't be able to manage us both. But now that it's gone, I'm sure I'll be okay.

Sam doesn't have a card like I do, so I've been assigned to take care of him—that is unless he continues on like he did a couple of nights ago. I went looking for him when he didn't come home from his night job. I found him drunk, wandering down the street. You see he's 82, and he's had to go back to work as a security guard to pay for his insurance. The church doesn't take care of him like they do me. The bishop came over the other night and brought all this food for us." He finishes his monologue and waves his hand around the neatly organized kitchen filled with jars of food.

John is a small frail man and wears wire-rimmed glasses. He has a warm smile and a cold handshake. I'm seeing him for end-stage colon cancer—the referral said uncontrolled pain, but obviously that's not a problem right now. John denies any need to see a social worker or a chaplain—that is "unless I can help someone else worse off than me."

During subsequent visits, I listen as John tells me of his childhood, marriage and of criminal charges made against him. "I did my time in prison for child abuse, but God and the church have forgiven me, so I know I'm going to heaven, especially with that ticket I showed you." He smiles almost smugly.

Not sure how to respond, but knowing I don't want to appear judgmental, I remain silent, and he continues. "I don't want to take any medications that might make me unable to take care of Sam in case he needs me. That's why I'm so happy to have my prayer answered about my pain."

"I'm glad the pain is gone, and I'll be able to help you deal with it if it does come back," I say.

"I don't want any medications around here. Sometimes my daughter comes to see me. She, or her boyfriend, might steal it to use or sell them. You see, she lives on the streets, but she comes over to get things from me or has me take her somewhere. I've tried to help her by taking her son in, but the law frowned on that, and now my grandson is a ward of the court. I think he's adopted by now and I can't even see him. You see it was my son that I abused, and now I can't be alone with any boys, even my own grandson." I am amazed at how open he is with me.

Though not outwardly expressive, I struggle internally. Part of me wants to shun him as a child molester. But when I set aside my personal opinions, I only see a man who is genuinely concerned for his family. There's no sense of apology from him for his actions. He blames the abuse on his wife's absence saying he was left alone with his kids. I can't deny the sadness within me, but I know he deserves the compassion I would give any dying person. Still my attitude changes slightly when he admits abusing his own son.

"But my son has forgiven me—he comes to see me often. He's important in the church," John says sounding proud and pleased.

John's brother Sam and his daughter Holly show up at my next visit, and I see the truth of his assessments. Indeed, Sam seems impaired in judgment and Holly looks hardened in her lifestyle. Sam can't grasp the seriousness of his brother's condition. Holly's only there to get money from her father. She is unable to make eye contact with me.

"NO Holly!" John emphatically repeats several times. "No, I can't give you any money." Denied a handout, Holly angrily slams the door.

Sam, as if he was reading his brother's mind, says, "No, you don't have to worry; I'm not going to go out and get drunk again. You took all my money so I can't." Sam turns to me, "My brother's not dying, is he? He just needs to exercise more, right?"

I say 'yes' to the question of dying and 'no' to the exercise. We discuss the seriousness of Sam being present for his brother. He agrees to help.

John calls the office three days in a row regarding his bowels. He's now asking me to help with his colostomy bag. Until now he's dealt with it himself. I give instructions over the phone. On the third day when he calls, I ask Sam if he'll be able to help because I can tell John is struggling to follow my directions. Sam responds, "Yes, but I can't help him with his colostomy bag. It came loose last night, and he has a mess all over the bathroom. I tried to help, but I can't stand it."

I hurry out to help, cleaning the bathroom and John up and changing the bag. I write out instructions in simple words so they both can understand them.

John accepts the medications when his pain returns with a vengeance. "I can't stand this. I'll need to keep any pills or liquid locked up so my daughter won't see them. She loves me and wants to help, but her addiction is stronger than her desire to help."

Realizing he can't manage alone he pleads, "Please call my son. Maybe he can come and talk to you. He won't let me see his boys, but I know he loves me and wants to help as much as he can." He hands a paper with his son Bill's number on it.

When I see Bill at the next visit, I see love in his eyes for his father. In front of John he states clearly, "No, my sister can't come and stay with him. She's not to be trusted. She'll only cause trouble for you, Dad," he says. "Isn't there some way we can help without using my sister? And you can't trust Sam either. He's messed up so many times, yet you always take him back, Dad. Why, I don't know."

I arrange for a meeting with a social worker, myself and John to problem-solve in the event he's unable to remain alone. I can see that Plan B will probably be needed in the near future.

The next week when I enter John's home I see he's noticeably upset. "This is the last picture I have of my grandson," John says through his tears. "I'd really like to see him one more time before I die. I want to give him a hug and wish him well in his life."

I am unable to succeed in getting him to see his grandson. When I reach the caseworker, I'm told that he can take a letter to the child, but he can't permit any personal contact. As I write John's words on the Easter card I've brought, my heart opens, and I feel very grateful to be helping him. Words of love pour out for this six-year-old grandchild. John knows this will be his last contact with him. Tears fill my eyes, and I have to wait for them to clear.

The next day, I find John lying on the floor. He has fallen on his way to the bathroom, and Sam is gone. "His Social Security check came, and he's out drinking," John whispers. I call John's daughter and the social worker, knowing I can't leave him alone.

I make John comfortable in his hospital bed in the living room. I'm able to leave when the social worker gets to the apartment. Besides watching John, she'll be busy making calls to arrange an urgent admission to a local nursing home.

Social Workers are such a godsend to us nurses, I think as I exit. *They really do rescue many a messed up situation.*

When I come back from another visit, John's daughter, her boyfriend and their Rottweiler are in his bedroom. Holly states that she won't approve moving her father into a facility. The social worker seems very grateful to see me.

This indeed is the worst challenge I've had. How many months until I retire? I ask myself.

Fortunately for all of us, John had us move the pain medication out of his bedroom so I don't need to intrude on their space.

When I call John's son Bill, we get permission to admit John to a nearby nursing home. Now we know he'll receive quality attention until he dies. He won't have to care for his family. Now his daughter can visit him but can't steal his medications.

When Bill arrives, I give him the teddy bear John wanted his grandson to have. He will later deliver it to the caseworker along with the Easter card.

Sam came to see his brother although the staff reported he was drunk, so was only allowed to be with John for minutes.

Peace at last, John!

Author's notes: Chapter 21
Ticket to Heaven

Note 1: Hospice personnel treat all people with respect and compassion without regard to an possible arrest record, their race or their religion. Treating all patients this way is especially important at end-of-life. I needed to set aside my feelings about John as a sex offender and give him compassionate care.

Note 2: I write the instructions out for John and his family but also for any nurses that might follow me on a day off or for a nurse who may be called during the night.

PART SIX

In-Facility Care

TIM AND HAPPY ROAD

Pushing open the squeaky gate that has "Happy Road Adult Foster Home" painted in big letters, I wonder what is in store for me. My peers have warned me about Tim. Every new client is different with different needs.

Elena, the Romanian caregiver, greets me. A very emaciated man stands next to her. She shakes my hand and says, "This is Tim, the one you are here to see."

Tim, as if responding to my thoughts of weight loss, quickly adds, "I'm so skinny because they don't feed me. When they do give me a meal, it's always cold. They won't give me what I want!"

Elena answers simply, "We try to give you what you want. You have a very poor appetite. And you've only been here a week." She welcomes me into her house—which is obviously a family home converted to a facility with small rooms for six residents. She shows me around and points to a sign that says Ring Bell If You Need Help. "We're glad you're here for Tim. We love working with hospice. I'm sure you'll help him a lot. Please remember to check in before you leave so you can sign our book."

Tim at 45 looks over 60. He has long, straggly, grey-brown hair and an unkempt salt-and-pepper beard. Skin hangs loosely on his six foot frame. His cheekbones stand out, and the area behind his eyebrows is sunken.

Tim invites me into his room. We walk down a narrow hallway past a small bedroom and tiny bathroom shared by residents who are able to walk. His room is around the corner.

This adult foster home accommodates patients with scant resources. Though modest, such homes are often an improvement, especially for those like Tim, who have been living on the street. His room is small with little extra space after the equipment is in place. Next to his hospital bed is the commode which he offers as a chair. On the bed is the latest crossword puzzle, nearly completed. A stack of filled ones is nearby. Tim wears gray sweat pants and a food-stained sweatshirt. His tennis shoes are dirty and he uses them as slippers with the shoestrings untied.

When he sits on the bed and kicks his shoes off, I notice that his arms are so skinny I could easily close my thumb and index finger around one with room to spare.

"I don't know why this place is called Happy Road. There's nothing happy about it, and I really don't like it. Can you get me out of here? No, then, can you help me get out back to smoke? There's a gazebo where we can all smoke, but they don't want me to go alone." He pauses and winks at me. "I don't know why they won't let me go by myself unless it's because I left here with my scooter the other day without telling them." He wiggles off the bed onto his wheelchair with minimal help from me.

I guide his wheelchair as we go down the ramp and he points over to the 'scooter barn' where several Amigo electric wheelchairs are stored between uses by other residents.

As I push him under the covered area, I'm grateful I'm not allergic to cigarette smoke. Three residents are in the gazebo, and the air is filled with smoke. Butt-filled ashtrays add their aroma. I've learned to reserve judgment even on lung cancer patients like Tim. I figure there's no sense in trying to change them now.

"I was a logger once," Tim says as he lights up and takes a big puff of a Camel. "I worked in the hills of Alaska. We did helicopter logging. Believe it or not, I was a very strong man." He flexes his puny right arm exposing a tattoo. "In case you are wondering, that's the name of my daughter. And the entire name—Samantha—was tattooed there with a heart around it."

Unable to read anything but "S—a" because of the loose skin folds, I say nothing waiting for him to continue.

"God, I've really lost weight—'cause they're not feeding me. In the old days I could and would take on anybody and win. Now I've taken on Death and I can't win." He looks down at his shirt. I'm sure I see a tear which I choose to ignore.

After pushing his wheelchair back up the ramp, he announces defiantly, "I'm going out to McDonald's to get some real food. Then I'll stop for my favorite candy—I really like those Reese's Peanut Butter Cups, especially the ones with white chocolate." His smile reflects poor dental hygiene, and he has several decayed teeth in front.

I get the message that he's through with me, so I leave his room and stop by the owner's kitchen. Her husband and two small children are sitting at the table for lunch. Elena picks up one of the kids and greets me with the child resting on her hip.

Referring to Tim, she says, "At times he's very difficult to work with, but my husband and I try to give him what he wants. We make sure the food is warm, but by the time he gets to it, it is cold. Tim's a complainer, but you know, he is about three years younger than I am. We want to be a family for him. He has no one and was a heavy drug user, living on the street until he came here. He was diagnosed with lung cancer, maybe two weeks ago. I hope he'll be able to stay here until he dies. How long do you think that will be?"

"No one can give that answer. Not the doctor, not the oncologist and not the hospice nurse," I reply, thinking how it never fails that someone wants to pin me down with an approximate time. "When I started this job, a crystal ball wasn't issued with my hospice gear. But I know that he won't live another year, probably not even six months."

"As for his complaining—many people need to complain. He has so little control of his life and since this is a recent diagnosis, he's still adjusting to it. My theory is that complaining helps people to feel some measure of control—if it's not the food, frequently it's the home or the pain. But we'll be working together to get Tim's needs met."

Elena mentions his daughter, Samantha. "No one knows where she is and that's the way he wants it."

And so Elena and I begin working together to help Tim be as comfortable as possible. Though she and her family are always attentive, he continues to appear unhappy. Still he refuses relocation when it is offered. "No," he emphatically states, "I've gotten used to them. I know they care for me."

"Would you like to make contact with Samantha?" I ask one day, thinking I might have time to do some sleuthing to locate her before he dies.

"I don't ever want her to see me this way. Besides I have no idea where she is. She was such a beautiful girl." He falls into a memory trip of childhood happy times. "She'd crawl on my back, and we'd romp around the room playing horsey." Tears follow, then an abrupt, "No, I don't want her to see me like this. It's better for her to not know any of this." He pushes away a hug from me.

Two weeks later, I stop at a 7-11 for white chocolate Reese's Peanut Butter Cups. Tim is now unable to get out of bed without help, let alone go out on his scooter.

When I give him his candy he says, "I think I'll lie here and eat these before I go down for a smoke. I had a dream last night, and it scared me. There was this great big globe with hundreds of bright lights on it. I was trying to get to it, but felt afraid. What do you think it could have meant?"

Before I can respond he continues, "I think it was about finding my peace and you know what? Next time, I will go toward it." I help him into the wheelchair noting again how much weight he has lost in such a short time.

"Well, I did dream last night," he greets me on the next visit, "but this time, I dreamed I was dead. And when I woke up, I was shivering in a cold sweat. Do you think I'll be dying soon?"

As gently and honestly as possible, I offer my interpretation. "I wonder if this dream is not helping you accept what death will be for you. And yes, you're continuing to lose ground. And yes, I do think your death will happen soon." Sharing too much information, yet being realistic, is a challenge when I'm asked this question. He appears less frightened and quickly asks to go outside for a smoke.

Now that he is only able to eat a few bites because of difficulty swallowing, he's looking more emaciated. Often with addicts, it can be challenging to get pain control because most of them have developed a tolerance for even a large amount of drugs. Fortunately for Tim, we've been able to use the pump to get on top of his pain. The pump gives a base rate of medicine. He's able to self-dose when the pain breaks through. It's much like a pump used in hospitals for postoperative pain relief.

I bring a CD of peaceful music after we'd talked about his fears of the dream. Tim loves the music and comments on his native Indian heritage after hearing a song about the Great Spirit. "My family told me about the Trail of Tears, so this song gives me some peace," he says as we sit and listening. Leaving the CD playing, I lean over his bed to hug him goodbye.

"It is such a good job you're doing, Tim," I say noting his newfound peaceful nature, "this job of dying is a hard one."

"No," he replies, "no, your job of getting to know and love people and then watch them die. That is the hard job. Thank you for coming to be with me."

Shortly after, I receive a call from Elena, "Sharon, can you come quickly? Tim's not responding. I think he's dying right now."

As soon as I enter his room, Tim opens his eyes, smiles and goes into a calm sleep. I sit beside his bed, holding his hand, knowing there will be no family to sit in vigil with him. "It's okay, Tim. It's okay to go. Now is the time for you to reach for that light you saw in your dream. There's no need to struggle anymore. You are loved."

For the next three days, Tim is intermittently present in consciousness. His eyes appear unfocused at times. He's briefly alert and then confused.

When Elena asks about this, I say, "It's like there's an imaginary line drawn on the floor, and Tim is straddling it. This side is our world," I say, looking down and standing on a tile line. "And this side," I step over, "is the other world. Sometime he has both feet on this side and other times on the other side. In his time, he will be on the other side totally." I pause looking at him and then back at her. "Heartwork is being done," I say tapping my own heart area. "This is work between him and his maker—and it takes time—as much time as needed. And then he will let go."

"But what can I do now? I want to help him," Elena responds.

"Right now, all we can do is to moisten his lips, turn him for comfort and be present as we witness his experience. This heartwork is very private.

You and I have come a long way in this little room with Tim. Thank you, Elena, he feels your love."

Two nights later, while taking night call, I get a page to call Elena.

"Tim is dead," she says, "he died very peacefully. He must have known you were on call."

Author's notes: Chapter 22
Tim and Happy Road

Note 1: Tim had a caregiver who wanted to be doing something for him at his dying time. I explained to her that this was a time to sit with him and hold his hand if possible. It was not a time when other actions are helpful. This is the vigil, and it is a time for being not doing.

Note 2: Tim's dream was very helpful for me. It provided an opening that allowed me to talk about what he was looking forward to and what his fears might be. I would often begin a conversation by asking how he was doing in the heart—meaning emotionally, not physically.

Note 3: Tim drifts in and out of awareness and responsiveness. This is common but can be disturbing to family. The explanation given has been very useful to allay fears that a loved one is in pain. Caregivers watch for grimaces or moans as indicators of any pain.

This is Her Last Chance

"Her family has been told this is Mary Ann's last chance. If hospice can't help us here, then she will need to be moved," Stella, the director of the Assisted Care Facility tells me. "Mary Ann can no longer come down to the dining room for her meals. She's become quite irritable, not allowing staff to change her soiled Depends or even help her out of bed. We have a policy that everyone gets out of bed, gets dressed and comes to the dining area unless they're with you guys on hospice. We figure if they qualify for hospice they don't need to be forced to get up," Stella explains. She turns to a caregiver in the office and asks her to take me to Room 112.

I find Mary Ann with her back turned toward me. Her daughter Rae turns toward me and smiles. "I'm afraid I can't make her get up. She's getting to be real crotchety lady." Then to her mother, "Please, Mom get up. A nurse is here to see you."

"Go away," Mary Ann grumbles. "Go away."

Rose, the caregiver, steps up to the bed. "Let me help you get up." Her voice is soothing as she places her arm under Mary Ann's and helps her swing her feet over the side of the bed. "She's generally pretty good in the morning, at least for me. There you go, Mary Ann, into your favorite chair."

Mary Ann mutters a thank you under her breath just loud enough for me to hear.

I say engagingly, wearing my best smile, "It's so nice to meet you. What a great view you have. Look at those little sparrows. I love to watch them at home, especially when the squirrel comes in the feeder."

Mary Ann leans forward, attempts to stand up and starts yelling, "Help me, help me. Get me outta here."

Rose returns to care for her allowing me to step out of the room with her daughter. In the quiet, I can begin to ask her the admission questions. To qualify for hospice benefits, with an Alzheimer's diagnosis, certain criteria must be met. These criteria are necessary since the normal duration of Alzheimer's disease can be as long a six to eight years and there must be a six month prognosis to receive hospice services. In questioning Rae, I find Mary Ann does meet the criteria. She's lost twenty-five pounds in two months; she can't control her bowel and bladder and she's no longer able to walk or feed herself. She is not eating nor drinking except when forced. These recent changes in her function and the weight loss gives us the go-ahead to help.

She spits all her medications out at the staff and has even tried to bite them when they've tried to help. Her problem behavior increases in the evening or when she's moved around. If she would begin to improve or even stabilize in six months, consideration would be given to discharge her from hospice.

When her daughter and I return to her room, Mary Ann is calm, back again in bed and facing the wall. She grunts as Rae says goodbye. I sit with her just to let her know I'm there. Then I speak softly, "Mary Ann, you'll be seeing me at least once a week; does that sound okay? You don't have to talk unless you want to, but I'll be checking in to see if you're having any discomfort or need anything. I'll talk to the staff and then your daughter in case she needs anything from me. So I'll say goodbye for now."

There is no response.

When I examine her chart records, I find several antipsychotics have been used to no avail. Respiradol, Trazadone, Valium have all been tried and discontinued. Anti-depressants have also been prescribed in case depression is the cause of her behavior.

It appears Mary Ann's confusion began about six months ago. She would pull off her Depends and pee on the floor. She had periods of garbled speech and became combative. She had denied pain when the staff had questioned her, but I wondered if pain could be the explanation for her behavior problems.

Observing her over several visits, I found her grimacing when I helped her out of bed. I hear the staff reporting more outbursts of anger when getting her ready for bed. I order acetaminophen(Tylenol) to be given regularly at night. Possibly night pain is causing some behavior problems. Many Alzheimer folks are unable to express their pain verbally, so they act out instead.

"It's so much easier to get her clothes off and get her into bed now," Rose reports after the mild analgesics are started. "But, you know, she's has trouble swallowing those big pills. Could we get the same thing in liquid form? Maybe we could get the medication for her constipation that way too because she spit them out last night."

When I deliver the liquid meds, Rose asks, "Could we use the Tylenol at other times during the day. I see her holding her back whenever we move her around. And did you notice how her fingers are bent—she couldn't even hold a glass if she wanted to?" I schedule the Tylenol for four times per day, since expecting the staff to read her behavior as pain is asking too much. I know facilities prefer scheduling instead of educating multiple staff on the Alzheimer patient's needs.

Mary Ann continues to refuse food. But with encouragement, she takes the liquid Tylenol occasionally. Rose notes on the days she refuses the Tylenol, her behavior worsens. She bent a caregiver's finger back while having her Depends changed just before I arrived for a visit.

I receive a call from the facility supervisor, "I know you're working with us on these behavior issues, but something more has to be done. I can't have my people injured by a resident. I'm going to have to call her daughter and give her the news. She needs to find another place for her mother…that is unless you have any ideas?"

"Yes, I do," I reply. "Before you call family, let me get her doctor's approval for Fentanyl, the pain patch. We can get this in a low dose. It might relieve her pain which I think is the reason for her bad behavior. You and your staff say she had a great personality before this acting out started. You and I both know that patients with dementia or Alzheimer are often unable to express their needs. But they can show us they're in pain. Remember that scale I showed you for dementia patients? I'll go over it with you the next visit I make if you like. Let me call Rae and talk with her. It's worth a try,at least. I hope we don't have to move her. You guys are so great with her."

175

When I call, Rae immediately praises hospice. "I'm so glad to hear your voice and I'm grateful you were called in. Mom actually smiled at me the other day. Hospice is great," she says before I tell her our latest concerns.

"Here's what's up with your mother," I say, pausing a moment to decide if I should mention the supervisor's threat, "I think your mother is having more pain than she's able to tell us. Alzheimer patients are unable to express themselves so we have to watch their actions, their facial movement or groans. Mary Ann seems to do better when the Tylenol is on board. The staff tell me she's not swallowing the Tylenol for her arthritis pain, so her relief is intermittent. I'd like to start her on a patch that releases medicine twenty-four hours a day. She wouldn't need to swallow this since it's a patch. It would be a small dose so she won't sleep all the time. I think she'd improve with this. If you're game, I'll get an order from her doctor."

When I deliver the patch, I apply it immediately without attempting to explain it to Mary Ann as her understanding is limited. Rose lifts Mary Ann's shirt, and I apply the tiny patch to her back where she won't be able to reach it.

"This will make you feel better, Mary Ann," I explain to her. Then to Rose, "Please tell your staff to note inappropriate behaviors. It'll take a while for the medication to take effect, and it will last for seventy-two hours. I'll bring more patches if she gets relief."

"You won't believe how much better Mary Ann is," the supervisor reports as I enter the next day. She lets the staff change her and get her up in her chair. She got a shower today."

When I walk into her room, I'm amazed at the smile I'm given. She's only able to say a few words, but her smile speaks volumes. A staff nurse is combing Mary Ann's hair without complaints. Mary Ann says, "Thank you." I'm sure that was meant for the caregiver, but I can also feel the gratitude down deep.

As I'm driving to her next visit, I'm reminded that Rae told me how Mary Ann used to love going out for a Burgerville shake. Impulsively I stop at the drive-thru and order a seasonal raspberry shake. As I give it to Mary Ann, a gleam appears in her eyes which melts my heart. She's only able to take a couple of swallows, but that was enough to fill me with happiness.

Mary Ann continues to exhibit a more pleasant behavior but refuses to eat. She also remains in the bed. The staff report how they're able to give her good care without any protests. Her daughter has called me to express her gratitude for making her comfortable. She states she's had some quality time sitting reading to Mary Ann or just being there.

I find out Mary Ann dies over the weekend. Rose calls me the next day and thanks me for making it possible for Mary Ann to remain with them rather than being sent to a memory care facility. "She needed to be here with her friends. And we needed her also."

I've learned a few things about pain over the years and the biggest thing is that when in pain no one can be nice.

Author's notes: Chapter 23
This is Her Last Chance

Note 1: Mary Ann had pain that was difficult to express or describe. This is often the case with dementia or Alzheimer patients. Facilities have a rapid staff turnover so they may not have the experience to discern pain because of the patient's behavior problems. Hospice nurses use a pain scale different than that of the 1-10 scale. We use body language, expressions and movement to rate pain for these patients.

Note 2: Mary Ann refuses to eat but suffers no pain. At this stage in her life eating is not important, and she will not feel hunger nor discomfort. Families are often afraid their loved one will hurt if not forced to eat. I've seen a calm come over these patients when nobody forces a spoon in their mouth.

"I know my mom likes to talk to you, so I'm not going to fire you, but I wish you didn't talk about dying so much. Mom says it disturbs her." Marcia has stopped me in the hallway outside her mother's room in the assisted living facility. "My sister and I disagree on what to do next, but we do agree on helping Mom live longer. So we'd like to have a conference with you. The nurse here is presenting Mom's case next week. Could you come on Tuesday?"

I check in with the staff regarding Ethel's routine care review. The RN in the facility coordinates the patient, family and caregiver's needs when hospice is not involved, so now she is happy to include me in the meeting.

"Ethel has been telling the staff she's going to die this weekend and that she's tired of being here. She also talks about going to the family cabin," I say to the group which consists of Ethel's two daughters and the facility RN. We are gathered in the conference room. Ethel will be brought in after the family concerns have been aired.

Anger, sadness and resentment erupt from her daughters. They seem to play tag-team in their comments about what their mother needs:

"If only she would eat more, she would live longer."

"If only she would walk more."

"If only she had an antidepressant."

"If only she could get a new hair style or be given a bath."

The most out-spoken one, Marcia, says, "We don't believe she really means what she's saying about dying. We think she wants to live and go to our cabin. Mom tells each of us different things. Then she says other things to the caregivers and to the hospice nurse."

I sense each daughter is caught up in her own agenda but realize that each is doing what she feels is best for their mother. I explain that Ethel's process is happening with or without permission of anyone. I say, "You've both seen how tired she is and how she just wants to be left alone. Sometimes she refuses to get out of bed or eat the meals served her. I know from experience that patients often lead their family on and try to please them. I think she could be trying to shield you from her true feelings. Maybe she feels able to share them with me and other caregivers without being corrected or hurting your feelings."

Marcia and her sister nod in unison. "I guess I get it," Marcia exclaims. "Maybe that's why she says all that to the staff and then tells us she wants to go to the cabin in Bend. Can we bring Mom in now? I'd like to hear what she has to say."

The RN gets Ethel who is sitting slouched down in the wheelchair. The first thing she says is, "I'm so tired. Can I go back to bed?"

I recognize a growing acceptance in the daughters' faces. "It's okay, Mom. We'll get you back to bed." Marcia stands up to push her mother back to her room. A caregiver meets them to help get Ethel into bed.

When Marcia returns, she says, "Yes, you're right. She is very tired. We know now that she is close to death. We didn't want to say it, but we both wanted to find a reason for her 'giving up.' I understand now," she says turning toward her sister. "Do you agree, Diane?"

Diane has been spending more time with her mother and has commented on how tired Ethel has been agrees. "Let's let her do it her way then. Thank you for meeting with us."

"You're most welcome, but you two did all the work. You just wanted to do all you could, so there'd be no reason to feel you hadn't done enough. This is very normal. All of us, including the staff here, will work to allow her to do the things she wants to do. She may not want to get out of bed anymore, but if she does, her wishes will be followed. If she only takes sips or bites of food, that'll be okay. Is that right?"

Tears are falling as they agree. I give them each a resource book, _Final Gifts_ by Maggie O'Callahan, as I hug and thank them for listening.

After the conference the rest of the family comes to see her and are able to tell her that they'll be okay. They now know she is actually ready to let go. They know there'll be no visit to the cabin—Ethel won't even get out of bed again.

"You know," Ethel tells me on the next visit, "my favorite grandson came to see me and told me that I didn't need to be in my body for him to feel my presence."

As she starts to cry I blink away my own tears. Then through our tears we truly see each other and can smile.

The daughters sit by her bedside day and night giving her what she needs or just holding her hand.

At her death, there is a true celebration though everyone is grieving. They know they have done all they could including letting her go. They've honored Ethel in allowing her to do it her way.

Author's notes: Chapter 24
The Same Page

Note 1: Ethel's family was familiar with case conferences. Facilities have them regularly to discuss changes in patient needs and any problems the family is having. These facilities usually welcome the hospice input because we have more time to spend with the patient and family than their staff does.

Note 2: "Letting go" was interpreted by her daughters as telling Ethel that she could die. This family was struggling with giving her permission, fearing it might be misinterpreted by their mother. In time they were able to tell her that they would miss her but that it would be alright if she felt she could die. Families often do not understand the difference between the need to fight for life and the need at some point to surrender to the flow of life and death. I believe this family originally wanted Ethel to fight.

Laughing Sally Faces Death

Sally lives in a non-traditional residential care facility with eleven other Medicaid folks. I mean non-traditional in a good way, since the caregivers here are full of heart providing good care without the expensive facade of many private pay facilities. Most of the residents here are alone, unable to care for themselves and dependent on the health-care system. Some have been on the streets or were alcoholics or addicts placed here by social workers. Other nurses from my agency have been here before and are very critical about the appearance. Outside and inside, the structure is run-down, and the rooms are small. But the staff truly cares about each person. Goats are pastured in a fenced area right next to the railroad. A river flows along the other side of the property and the residents are restricted from access by a fence and gate.

As I arrive to visit Sally, I see a table under a covered area with smoke rising up from each of the five people sitting there. A man stands up, smiles and extends his hand, introducing himself as Pat, the owner. His wife is on the left with two older men, and across from them sits an older blonde female with dark roots showing. In the center are three butt-filled ashtrays with ashes overflowing. One of the older gentlemen makes a wolf-whistle at me, and Pat shushes him. A couple of Chihuahuas are yapping under the table with one walking around on her front legs.

Intrigued, I introduce myself and ask about the dog.

Pat explains, "Oh, Ollie runs around like that when it's been raining because she can't stand water on her hind legs." Everyone at the table starts laughing.

One curmudgeon shows a toothless grin and says, "I can tell we're going to have fun with you."

Pat introduces the other folks at the table, "This here is Andy, Sandi and Bob. And you're here to see Sally, right?

"Bob was just discharged from hospice since he was doing so well. I'm sure glad it's you coming to care for her. You came here several years ago; I think it was a diabetic you saw then, but you probably don't remember."

In that moment I do remember how judgmental I was way back then though I was quickly won over by the excellent care at his facility. I know Sally, an end-stage breast cancer patient, is in good hands here.

Pat shares Sally's story when he's out of earshot from others. "When Sally first came to us, she was really down and out. She'd been kicked out on the street by a man she lived with. He was beating up on her. She has two daughters who refuse to bring their kids to visit since she's so difficult. Before she got bed-bound, she was constantly looking for drugs and alcohol, trying smuggle them in here. But I'd always find them." He opens the door to the common area revealing dining tables covered in oilcloth with artificial flowers in the center of each. "I worry about hospice coming in because I know, regardless of how many drugs you give her, she'll want more. She's always asking for her Vicodin. We have to crush it and give it to her in food because she's had difficulty swallowing with the tracheostomy. She had to have that after the radiation. She's difficult to care for—complaining all the time, refusing to allow us to change her bed or bathe her—that's why her grandchildren can't come and visit her."

I look around when we enter the TV room. It has twelve chairs lined up against the wall. The furniture appears functional, but not modern or fancy. I see a caregiver kindly speaking to a resident about going to the bathroom. She appears polite in her exchange with an older deaf woman. For a moment, I think how the admission nurse and the supervisor thought I would be an excellent nurse for this patient even though other nurses had found working here difficult.

"Sally's room is over here," Pat interrupts my thoughts as we climb the stairs to an upper level. Sally's room is packed with medical equipment: hospital bed, oxygen concentrator, bedside table, suction machine with boxes of disposable kits to suction the tracheostomy and a big television set.

The bed is piled high with coloring books, loose crayons, Fig Newtons, Oreos, puzzle books and a large amplifier which looks like a microphone. The bare light bulb's string is tied to the over-the-bed-table.

Sally's first comment explains the state of her bed: "I need all these things here so I can reach them." She grabs the amplifier which I'd mistaken for a microphone and holds it to her neck. The tracheostomy was done six months ago along with a laryngectomy. Now she needs the amplifier to be heard.

She looks up at me and smiles. "Hi, I'm glad to see you. I've heard a lot about you from the other nurse." Sally's only three months older than I am but looks years my senior. Her thin face is framed with long, stringy, matted, black hair. She wears a seersucker dress with food stains covering the tiny flowers in the design. Her fingernails are two inches long, stained and dirty. "The first nurse said I'd like you because you're real funny. I like to laugh and play. Pat, can you suction me now? He's the only one I trust to do it since one of the caregivers almost killed me—taking so long to get me clear of the mucus." She speaks quickly as he turns the machine on, knowing her breathing is blocked while he suctions her tracheostomy.

When he finishes, she says, "See my coloring books?" She holds up a neatly colored page featuring Strawberry Shortcake. "I do this while I'm watching the country western channel when I can't sleep."

I comment on the stack of completed coloring books.

Sally continues in a rambling style, "I asked my daughter Wendy to buy some of those sparkling crayons, but she hasn't done it yet." She turns to Pat smiling. "He's willing to sit with me at night if I'm scared." And to him she says, "You are a great caregiver. Thank you." Pat smiles and leaves the room.

I question Sally about the pictures that cover the walls and she responds, "That's my Momma and that's my granddaughter, Etta. She's two. The other one is my grandson, Ben, who's eight. I haven't seen them in a long time. Can you fix my pillows, please? And raise my bed? The remote's over there."

"You know Sally, I could use this control to raise your head...but watch out, I might raise it enough to dump you in the river." I'm smiling so she knows I'm only kidding.

185

"You know," she laughs, "I like you. I want you to come back."

I reach to get closer and nearly choke myself on that light bulb string tied to her bedside table. I apologize, and she laughs again. "I'll tell you right now, anybody coming to see me has got to know how to laugh. Wanna watch Judge Judy with me? She makes me laugh and I laugh at anything funny."

She turns her attention to the TV and waits for a commercial to answer my question about her pain.

"Yes, I have a lot of pain, mostly in my legs. That pill doesn't always help so I ask for more. They don't like me asking for so much of it, but it hurts."

She answers my question about the use of a pain patch. "Yes, I'd try it if it could help. I want you to know that I don't want to be sleeping all the time. I have to do my puzzles and my coloring books."

With each visit I try to balance her physical needs with what she will permit from those she allows to care for her. She says, "I hope you're okay with the fact that I asked that social worker not to come again. She doesn't even crack a smile. I can't have that." She looks at me as if she wants my approval. "I know I'm dying, but I don't want people to be morose about it."

Then one day she surprises me with, "All right, you convinced me; I'll have one of those people who give baths come in, but she can't wash my hair or cut my nails. I'm afraid of drowning when she washes my hair. Water got into my trach one time. And you don't know how long it took me to grow these nails. I can't let her cut them off!"

The very next visit, I meet the hospice aide as she finishes her assignment. Sally says, "She is good—did you know that? And she washed and cut my hair. I'll bet you didn't know she's a hairdresser?" She appears pleased with herself, her eyes sparkling with delight and laughter. "And I let her file my nails. She can polish them but never cut them."

Amazing what a little pain control can do to improve attitude.

Excitedly, Sally tells me that her grandchildren came to visit her. "Etta's so cute and smart. She had on this darling little outfit, and she sang for me. Ben's quiet, but he liked coloring in my book. It's so nice to see them."

On my way out Pat stops me. "This is a major change— both daughters are bringing their kids and spending time with her. Hospice has made a big improvement. Sally is back to her friendly cheerful self. I haven't told you the story of the day she arrived here, have I? The day I admitted her, she showed me this black breast looking like coffee grounds and said it was very hard. I got scared. I got her to the doctor the next day, and the following day she was in surgery for a mastectomy. Chemotherapy followed, and then she had to have a tracheostomy done after the radiation burned her throat. She's had a rough go. I'm glad you are helping her. She's a good lady."

Today Sally looks good; her bed is clean and she has bright red nail polish on her fingernails and a smile on her face: "Did you meet Bob? He was fired from hospice because he wasn't dying quick enough. Well, we have become good friends—he's like a boyfriend, and I want to go downstairs and sit next to him in our wheelchairs. Do you think that's possible?" Her eyes sparkle. "Pat got us some walkie-talkies, and we talk when we can't sleep at night. We tell jokes and laugh. I think he likes me." Pain and dizziness have prevented Sally from being comfortable being out of bed, but I think this is might be a good thing for her to try.

"Go for it," I reply.

"Look at this," she holds up a brightly colored picture in her coloring book. "I think it looks like you. Would you like it?" She rips the page and offers it to me—it is a girl wearing hiking clothes and boots.

I take it, thanking her, reminded of the times I have shared stories of my hiking trips up the Columbia River Gorge.

"I'm trying to do a page for each person in my family. This one is for Bob. It's bright red roses, just like he brought in for me." She nods her head toward a vase with a now wilted arrangement of roses. "He told me that he wasn't going to let me die. I've never felt love like this before."

But as her pain increases, so do the pain medications, though her spirits remain positive and cheerful. "My grandkids, Etta and Ben, came yesterday, and we all sat here and did coloring. It was fun—they didn't want to go home. I sure love those kids. I'm getting ready for Christmas by ordering presents from these catalogs," she says, holding up four catalogs with items circled.

"Growing up my life was pretty sad, but I was always laughing. In order to tell me from my cousin Sally, my family started calling me Laughing Sally, and it has stuck." She smiles, "I haven't always been laughing though. I had a tough life on the ranch with an alcoholic husband who beat me. I started drinking and didn't stop until I came here. They've been so good to me in this place. Pat is the greatest. He runs a tight ship here."

I'd witnessed how he had earned her trust and knew she meant it.

I've increased my visits to twice a week. We sit and watch television, or I play my harmonica. Teasingly she says, "You aren't very good—but you are sincere!" We laugh much and often. "I couldn't sleep last night, so I lay here and colored these pages," Sally smiles as I look at the beautiful green grass with flowers surrounding it.

I think she's using these bright crayons to color her world beautiful and to fill the lonely hours.

"You know, I'd like to talk to my sister in Wyoming, but I can't use this cell phone and the amplifier—it buzzes too much."

I ask a speech therapist to come to help, and he solves the problem by bringing out a device that blocks the extra noise. "Now I am able to call my daughters on their phones and tell them what I want. It'll be so nice to talk to my sister and let her relay to my father since he can't hear on the phone."

Sally wants to have a celebration before Christmas. "Maybe even a toast— you know I used to drink. Maybe we could have champagne. Let's talk to Pat about it. I'm sure he wouldn't mind, and I'll bet he has glasses we can use."

At each visit, I notice items arriving for her Christmas presents. She is excited about the coming party. No one but Sally knows which present is for whom.

"I love keeping secrets. Can you help me wrap these?"

I offer to get a volunteer to help and even provide a Santa Claus the agency uses each year.

She answers quickly, "That would be so great. I never saw Santa when I was a kid and never took my kids to one. Yes, please, please, please."

One day soon after that, I am requested to make an extra visit. Pat says, 'My caregivers thought she was dead—she didn't answer when they called, and she felt cold when I touched her. She's still alive, but I think she's dying."

Sadness comes over me, because I hadn't had enough time to prepare her family or have the celebration, but when I get there she rallies and smiles and says, "I'm ready to stop all my medications. I am tired of this. I was floating over my bed. I heard Pat ask me if I was cold and I remember saying that I wasn't because where I was at that moment I wasn't. I don't want anything more to eat. I'm ready to go!" Then the very next day, when she tells the staff she's hungry, we start the food and the medications again.

When I check in with Pat the next visit, he says anxiously, "These spells of being cold, of not responding for hours, are happening every night. One night, her hand dangled off the bed; we put it back up there and it fell off again—we couldn't move her over to the center of the bed because she was such dead weight. I think she is close to death!"

Sally, on the other hand, doesn't think much of these spells and says, "Just tell them not to worry about it unless I am really dead and then they won't need to even think about me because I'll be gone."

I often see folks who rally after a marked decline, and I consider these as "dress rehearsals." I mention to her that with the increasing occurrence of these spells, I need to tell her daughters, but I hear only resistance.

She says, "I'm not leaving just yet. This is far too lovely a world to leave now. I feel love like I've never felt and don't want to leave it." She allows me to call only one of her daughters.

From this moment on, only gratitude, laughter and acceptance are heard in every conversation. She intends to get the coloring books completed. Grandchildren come much more frequently.

One day while I'm visiting, Etta enters wearing a beautiful little purple velvet dress. She jumps up on the bed, gives Sally a kiss and says, "Love you, Grammy." Little Ben is very quiet but intent on coloring. "Can we start right now?" He's well dressed in a cute cowboy shirt and boots.

The children's mother says later that healing occurred during these sessions. "She never colored when she was little and neither did we. There was a lot of connection when we did this. As she told us why she chose violet for this or red for that, my kids got a chance to get to know their grandmother. I am so glad we did this with her. I'm so grateful hospice was able to give our mother back to us."

After the family leaves, Sally relates an important dream. "I saw my mother shaking the bed. She told me it was time for me to come with her. I'm okay with that, but please don't tell my family—not yet anyway."

My heart opens and a tear falls, unnoticed except by me.

Several days later, arriving for a visit, I get no response from Sally as I call her name.

Is she floating above her bed again?

As I am about to leave the room, Sally speaks, "I was running on the beach, playing with my kids. It was so beautiful."

"I need to tell both your daughters. They have a right to know what's happening."

"Okay, I guess you're right. And tell them about the gathering we're planning. Make sure they know I want a drink—maybe I should have two or three. Tell them Jack Daniels is my favorite."

The very next day, Pat calls, "Sharon, she's not responding and she needs suctioning at least every five minutes. I want you to come quickly. Her family will be here any minute."

When I get to the care center, her second daughter who's been having trouble accepting the process, has just left. She's planning to return after taking her child to school. Etta, Ben and their mother are just going into Sally's room.

"Grammy, Grammy, wake up. Grammy, wake up it's me. It's Etta. Please wake up and talk to me," I hear this plea as I walk into the room.

I take Etta's tiny hand at her mother's request and walk out to see the pygmy goats. Ben comes too, "so Mom can have some quiet time with Grammy," he says. Etta's hair's in two little pigtails, and she's wearing a cute outfit of matching shirt and pants.

Ben calls my attention to a train going by—acting like he knows was going on. "My Grammy's not going to be here long, is she?" He asks.

I nod my head.

When I go back, Sally is mouthing, "I love you" to her daughter. I lean down and kiss her on the forehead, silently thanking her for the privilege of accompanying her thus far and wishing her well on her journey. She didn't get the presents labeled nor did she get her celebration—at least not in this lifetime.

Author's notes: Chapter 25
Laughing Sally Faces Death

Note 1: I was able to see the facility Sally was in really cared for her. She had definitely learned to trust the providers, so I knew I needed to work closely with them.

Note 2: Sally had visions before her death. This isn't unusual, and I used them to help guide the staff and myself.

Note 3: There is often a rally before death. I call it a practice run or dress rehearsal—to check out how it will work—perhaps. When Sally didn't die after she stopped eating, she realized it wasn't her time, and she began eating again.

"Oh, you are so going to love her," Debbie says as I ask about Priscilla, my next hospice patient at the assisted living facility. "She thinks she is the cat's meow. Wait until you see her." Debbie is one of the finest, most compassionate caregivers here, so I think if she likes Priscilla, I will also. Over the years I've often worked with Debbie, and we've shared the love of many residents who have been put on hospice. Debbie continues describing Priscilla, "She sits there in the middle of this huge queen size bed in jacquard-patterned silk pajamas telling everyone what to do."

I know I'm in for quite an experience when I visit her. Priscilla, a frail 110 pounds, has the most exquisitely dyed blond beehive hairstyle I've ever seen. She looks younger than her 86 years in her silk jacquard pajama top and bottom. And indeed, she does appear to reign over her "court" from the center of a very messy queen-size cherry wood poster bed. She has a beautiful white Persian cat lounging on her lap.

"Meet Baby, she is my best friend. I've had her since she was a little kitten. She'll greet you every visit." This cat is so perfect that she could easily have been the model for the large ceramic feline figurine Priscilla uses as a door stop. Baby is "kneading bread" on her mistress' chest while gazing at me with the most amazing blue eyes.

Even in the bed, Priscilla carries the grace of a very elegant and wealthy lady. I recognize her as a resident I've often seen being pushed in her wheelchair to the dining room. She always dresses to the nines with matching jewelry, watch, earrings and stylish clothes. Now as she looks me over, her comment is, "Yes, I like your pants. You can trade yours for a pair of mine when you leave—yes, they will fit me just fine." I gaze toward the open closet door which is full of elegant garments. "I love my clothes, especially the bright ones. I go shopping at Macy's as often as I can. Now

I can only get out once a month for my hair appointment—so I don't get to shop very often," she says, pausing to finger her hair.

"It is very hard just to make it to that appointment, but it's the most important thing for me and only one stylist can do it right. I have worn my hair like this since I was married, the first time—see that picture over there." She points to a portrait of herself as a lovely smiling 30-year-old with same hairstyle. "I only have to have it done every four weeks—she does it so well that I do nothing in between appointments. I can't sleep lying down because I can't breathe that way, so my hair stays perfect."

My ears perk up when she says she can't sleep flat but uses four pillows to prop herself up so she can breathe. This symptom is expected with a diagnosis of congestive heart failure. Along with this is a big decrease in energy so it is difficult for her to go out or participate in activities in the building. Her referral to hospice is due to a recent hospital stay for her heart condition.

Priscilla's financial support is depleted and application for Medicaid is being made. With hospice support of increased visits and personnel resources, she'll be able to remain in this Assisted Living Facility.

She tells me, "You know, my last husband had a lot of money. He bought me five new Cadillacs over five years. We had a home at Otter Crest and Lawrence Welk came to visit there often. And just look at me now. It is amazing how quickly money comes and money goes," she says with a twinkle in her eyes. "Judy is a friend and caregiver that I used to pay handsomely. She said she'll still come regularly even if I can't pay her a lot. She takes me to my hairdresser. I think she's doing this because she loves me so much!" A smile lights her face. "You'll meet her soon. She comes every day and stays until two o'clock. She's not spending as much time with me now that she has a housemate. I don't know what she sees in him—except maybe his money."

What a hoot, I think as I leave her room. We'll have a good time. With her spunk, she's not going to give up—I like that in a hospice patient. I'm sure I'll be like that. I bet she is going to control this whole process like a director in a movie.

The very next visit, I meet Judy. I find her attentive and pleasant yet also very controlling. She has been with Priscilla through two marriages and deaths, starting out as friends before she became her caretaker.

"I clean her apartment as much as she lets me. I shop for her, take care of Baby and buy her much-loved Coke. I also take her to the beauty shop—that's getting very difficult because of her weakness and shortness of breath," Judy explains her role. "She gets testy sometimes when I'm not here as long as she wants, but I'm here for three hours a day during the week. She sleeps most of the time I'm here with her," she says just as if Priscilla wasn't listening.

The subject of the conversation interrupts, "I do not. You won't talk to me. You just want to go home to that man. I don't know what you see in him except maybe his money!" The relationship between these two women seems complicated, at times adversarial, sometimes loving, then mother-daughterly; at times as an employer or hired help.

"She sleeps too much. Don't you dare give her more morphine; I've heard hospice nurses are liberal with morphine. If you give it to her, she'll just sleep a lot more and never eat. I try to bring her things from home, but she's just not hungry," Judy says to me. "You know she has that patch on for the pain in her back, don't you? Isn't that enough morphine?" Judy asks.

Priscilla explains, "I had a pain pump put in my stomach up at OHSU for back pain years ago, but it doesn't work now. Can you take it out? It takes up space and limits my breathing. The patch for the back pain is changed every three days."

"Yes, I know about the patch, and no, I can't remove the pump. You would need to go back up to OHSU," I explain only to be interrupted.

"They won't do it." Priscilla speaks up, "They say I wouldn't make it through the procedure—but I'm fooling them and everybody else. I'm going to be dancing at one hundred years old. So, watch out, world!"

On the next visit, Priscilla complains about sliding off her four pillows and ending up on the floor. She shows me her bruises.

"I can get a hospital bed, but we'll have to—," I start and she immediately holds up her hand.

"Shush! Don't even think about it. I will never be in a hospital bed. This here's my office, my dining room and my living room. I keep everything right where I can reach it. NO hospital bed," she says.

Indeed, this bed is her office with everything she needs on it. Whether or not she could find what she wants is another story. She has letters, stamps, bills and newspaper ads mixed in with her cat's toys and last year's Christmas candy. Judy tries to clean up things in the room—but no go.

"I won't move that thing. Someone might steal it," Priscilla says, pointing to the electric wheelchair, "if I put it in the hall." In order to get to the bathroom, she has to weave her way through stacks of magazines, a sewing machine and the electric wheelchair. She squeezes along the bedside using the soft mattress to support her until she reaches her walker.

"I plan to use the sewing machine to make quilts and I just might want to read those magazines," she declares. "These things are the only connection I have with my grandkids, so they have to stay here where I can see them," Priscilla says, almost defiantly, picking up a glass pig. After admiring it, she offers me a piece of chocolate from a See's candy box.

Judy finds a way to give love and be present in spite of all the negative comments between them. I'm amazed and impressed at this. She appears compassionate yet able to rebut derogatory comments—these comments, I think are spicing up an otherwise boring and somewhat depressing life for Priscilla.

When conversation leads in the direction of death or dying, Priscilla is adamant, "I am going to live to be 100 and dance at my party." She comments about my friend who had died just before the last visit, "Your friend Bill would not have died at 60 if I had known him, I'd have had him dancing with me. I've had so much fun, and it is not over, but why do we end up talking about death, anyway? And why don't you come more often? Can I call the office and tell them I need you two times a week?"

"Yes, you could do that, but it won't work unless you actually need the visit."

With noted deterioration, I begin to offer changes that might make her life easier, some of which she accepts, while others she vehemently rejects.

The facility calls the office on a day off so another nurse sees Priscilla and orders oxygen since she complained of increased shortness of breath.

"Get that damn stuff out of here! I don't have room for it and I won't use it," Priscilla screams at me the very next day. "If you'd just get that damn box out of my belly, I'd have more room to breathe, and everything'd be all right."

With her increasing tiredness, difficulty getting to and from the bathroom and the struggling to carry on a conversation, I know the disease is progressing. When she has a very low blood pressure reading, I suggest decreasing some medicines which might improve her energy level.

Her response is, "If it ain't broke, don't try to fix it. I am getting along fine—and don't bring that oxygen back in here." Feeling a little frustrated with her I comply with her wish.

Her cat is the center of her universe. Most of what she talks about is Baby. One day I arrive to find her upset. "This place has a new nurse, and she asked whether Baby is mine. She said she had a cat that looked just like Baby, and it had recently run away. I think she thought I had taken her cat—that's just not right. Baby has always been mine. Please tell me she can't do that. She can't take my Baby—can she?"

"No," I reassured her. Then I think this is a perfect lead-in for me to ask if she has thought who would get her precious friend when she died.

"Well," she admits, "I have thought about it. One of my daughters said she would take her, but she has a dog. Baby has never been outside my room, let alone seen a dog, so yes, I am worried. Will you take her? Oh, that's right you have a dog too."

So, I promise her that every effort will be made for Baby to get a good home. Judy plans to interview people to adopt Baby.

Before the next visit, I get a little calico kitten myself. Priscilla delights in hearing stories about her pranks. She relates, "When Baby was a kitten she slept in the sink. See here, I have a photo of her. Even now she jumps up on my lap while I'm sitting on the toilet and lets me comb her long white hair."

Even though her energy is decreasing, Priscilla's sense of humor never falters. The next visit as I am leaving, out of nowhere she asks, "Have you found me the man you promised?" We had talked about men, her husbands, my husband and men in general, but never had I made such a promise to her. I know she has something on her mind so I take the bait.

"Well, you better hurry up, because I don't have much time, and I have a surprise for him, and I must be awake for that!" I'm already at her door, so I know this is a ploy to keep me talking. So I play along. "And what is this surprise?" I ask, recognizing this is the first time she's acknowledged her decline.

"Come closer," she whispers when I come back, "'cause I got it sewed up, and there is nowhere down there for him, and he will want to know how I had three kids and now have no place to put it!" I laugh so hard that I stay longer to compose myself. After all, I think, hospice nurses shouldn't be seen leaving a dying person's room laughing. What a character she is, outspoken, manipulative, judgmental, controlling— yet what a delight.

Two weeks later, Priscilla goes out for her beehive hairdo with nearly disastrous results due to her tiredness and inability to transfer to the stylist's chair. By now, she is taking small doses of morphine by mouth for breathing problems when needed, and Judy gives her a dose while she's out of the apartment with no reported change in her breathing difficulty. The stylist and Judy had trouble getting her back into the wheelchair.

Debbie calls the very next day, "Priscilla's having a lot of trouble— please come quickly. She's very confused. She keeps talking about a dog named Boo. I think she's been dreaming or hallucinating. We're worried." On arrival, I see that indeed Priscilla has changed and appears to be close to the active phase of dying. This phase usually lasts three to five days before death and always predicates a call to the family to tell them of the change.

When I call Nancy, the only daughter who remains in contact with her mother, she says "No, I don't think you should call my sisters—there have been lots of issues over the years." She finally consents when I tell her this might be a last opportunity for forgiveness for all involved. Evidently Priscilla had alienated her other daughters, but they both respond to Nancy's call. They bring husbands and grandchildren for a final visit with Grandma.

That afternoon, I find them circled around the bed with Priscilla not responding to anybody or anything. Out of nowhere, Baby jumps upon the bed, starts working her magic—kneading bread—on Priscilla's chest, and suddenly she arouses and looks around the room. "Well, thank you all for coming. Can I have some Coke?" Everyone exchanges looks virtually dropping their jaws. Then they turn to me wondering what this is all about.

"It happens sometimes," I tell the family when we step outside. " A rally often happens right before the end. I call it a dress rehearsal." A part of me thinks they blame me for being in cahoots with their mother to get them to visit. Smiling, I tell them, "I guess Baby has just given CPR—cat pulmonary resuscitation."

Back at the bedside I say to Priscilla, "I guess Baby's not ready to let you go yet."

Things return to near normal except for Priscilla's weakness. She appears alert and is willing to eat small bites of food. It now requires two people to transfer her to the commode. She relates the dream she had on the day she had so much trouble. "I guess the dream was really about me instead of my dog Boo—he was trapped one day long ago just like I was in that bathroom when Debbie found me. One thing you need know, I'm definitely not going to the hairdresser again. She nearly did me in. I have a black wig I'll wear when this hairdo goes flat."

I believe that Priscilla knows she's had this event as a false start, and the real performance is going to happen soon. She never again says she will live to be 100 and dance. From this point on, she is so exhausted that she is unable to get to the bathroom alone or even carry on a short conversation.

When I remind her of my retirement the next week she says, "Well, then, I guess I'm leaving, too. It really is time."

I firmly believe that our loved ones have some control over that final phase and indeed Priscilla is saying she wants me there for her. I feel some sadness with this.

I order a hospital bed (after Judy convinces her of its necessity). As soon as it is delivered, Priscilla injures her wrist trying to pull herself up into bed. I get a splint and wrap the wrist to immobilize it.

"I'm having so much pain," she says, "I'm hurting all over. Please help me."

I increase the pain and the anti-anxiety medications and instruct the staff who will replace me. Two days after my retirement, Priscilla dies peacefully. Baby is given to a man who interviewed with Priscilla when she was alert.

When I receive the call of her death, I remember giving Priscilla this quote and laughing with her about it. Now whenever I see it, I think of her:

"Life should NOT be a journey to the grave with the intention of arriving safely in an attractive, well preserved body, but rather to skid in sideways, chocolate in one hand, wine in the other—body thoroughly used up, worn out and screaming: WOO HOO-what a ride!"

Dance, Dance, Dance!

Author's notes: Chapter 26
Dancing at 100

Note 1: Several years before her admission to hospice, Priscilla had a pain pump inserted under the skin to treat her arthritis pain. This pump requires that the patient make appointments to refill the reservoir with medication which she had failed to do. Hospice did not make any arrangements for its removal or refilling since it would require clinic visits.

Note 2: I urged Priscilla to have equipment brought in such as a bed and oxygen. But she flatly refused until it was absolutely necessary.

Study Questions for
Whose Death Is It, Anyway?

As we travel through life and learn of the death of an acquaintance or know the deep pain when a loved one dies or reflect on our own mortality, at some point we begin to process how it might be for us. Reading these stories can provide a framework for either personal or group discussion. Be it your own reading or in a book group, the questions that follow can help start a dialogue about death with ourselves and with those who will be there for us when we die.

I suggest writing your answers down in a journal and sharing the answers with others who have read the book.

For other questions that may arise, for example on accessing an Advance Directive or where to find information about Death with Dignity, feel free to use the resources listed in this book.

> Has one of your friends or relatives died recently? How did you feel about that death?
>
> What is a good death?
>
> How would you envision your death? Who would you like to be with you?
>
> If you were told you had six months to live, how would you spend them?
>
> Have you expressed in writing what your final wishes are?

What is an Advance Directive? Where can you get one? Do you need one if you've told your family what you want?

Can you be assured that you will not suffer at your time of death?

What would you want your family to do if you were in a near fatal car crash, and your family is told you have a flat line EEG?

What about those eleven most important words? What are they, and how do you want to use them?

What do you say to your mother when she tells you she's tired of living and is no longer interested in eating?

Does refusing to eat cause pain?

How prepared are you for your parents' deaths or even your own?

Do you have any concerns about dying?

What are some ways you can prepare for death?

Did this book lend more understanding about hospice or the dying process?

Resources:

Graceful Passages: a Companion for Living and Dying
Michael Stiltwater and Gary Malkin. Book and CD set.

Final Gifts: Understanding the Special Awareness, Needs and Communications of the Dying
Maggie Callahan and Patricia Kelley – Bantam Books, 1992.

Anam Cara: A book of Celtic Wisdom,
John O'Donohue – Harper Perennial, 1998.

Call Me By My True Names: The Collected Poems of Thich Nhat Hanh
– Parallax Press, 1999.

The Four Things That Matter Most: A Book About Living
Ira Byock, M.D. – Free Press, 2004.

Compassion and Choices: End-of-Life Consultation Program
Its mission is to improve care and expand choices at the end of life. Offers information regarding state specific Advance Directives, Dementia Provision and Sectarian Health Care Directive.
http://www.compassionandchoices.org
Ph: 800-247-7421.

National Palliative Care and Hospice Organization
A charitable organization created in 1992 to broaden America's understanding of hospice through research and education. Information regarding hospice admission criteria and services available locally.
http://www.nhpco.org

ABOUT THE AUTHOR

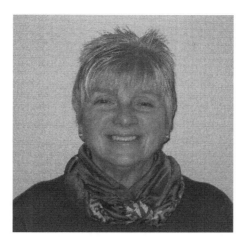

Sharon White has retired from a lifelong career as a registered nurse, spending forty years providing care and support to patients and their families. Her first exposure to death was when she was sent by an instructor in her first week of nursing school to the Los Angeles County General Hospital Morgue to complete an assignment on a man she had given care to the day before. As she stood in front of the huge cooler, the attendant pulled shrouded bodies, tray after tray, until the name of her patient appeared on the toe tag. The very next day she had a moderately ill woman as a patient who told her she would die at two o'clock that afternoon, and indeed she died right at the predicted time. These two moments brought her very close to her own mortality, and she continued dealing with the mystery of death throughout her career.

She became at ease with death and dying throughout her career, spending the last ten years of her career working with families and dying patients in their homes. She found people in the throes of the dying process to be great teachers and decided to journal about each death.

Sharon lives in Portland, Oregon with her husband Bruce, dog Ginger and cat Patches. She revels in the green of nature where she renews her spirit.

Contact: sharinjoy2003@hotmail.com

Made in the USA
San Bernardino, CA
31 March 2014